THE
BIPOLAR
GAME CHANGER

Harvest Your Special Messages, Glorify Your Superpowers
and Re-Uncover Your Mania to Level Up Your Life

Andrea Grey

Legal Disclaimer

By reading this book, you are agreeing to accept all parts of this Disclaimer. Thus, if you do not agree to the Disclaimer below, STOP now, and do not read this work.

For Educational and Informational Purposes Only.

The information provided in or through this book is for educational and informational purposes only and solely as a self-help tool for your own use.

Cover Design: sam_designs1

Book Interior Design: vaia creative + fiverr.com/tlmason

References: J.A. Rapps

Editing: Marie Still

Not Medical Advice.

The author and this work are not holding ourselves out to be doctors/physicians, psychiatrists, psychologists, therapists, counselors, social workers, nurses, physician's assistants, advance practice nurses, or any other medical professionals ("Medical Provider"). We are not providing health care or medical services. Although I have experience in helping myself and others with quality-of-life for bipolar, you agree and acknowledge to not consider the content of this work as medical advice in any way. Any specific concerns that you have about medications, herbs or supplements, and other medical concerns should be discussed with your medical provider. Do not disregard medical advice or delay seeking medical advice because of information that you have read in this book. Do not start or stop taking any medications without speaking to your own Medical Provider. If you have or suspect that you have a medical problem, contact your own Medical Provider promptly.

Personal Responsibility and Limitation of Liability.

You acknowledge that you are solely and personally responsible for your choices, actions, and results, now and in the future. You accept full responsibility for the consequences of your use, or non-use, of any information provided in or through this book, and you agree to use your own judgment and due diligence before implementing any idea, suggestion, or recommendation from this book to your life, family, or business. You understand that any recommendations are to be taken at your own risk, with no liability on my part, recognizing that there is a rare chance that illness, injury or even death could result, and you agree to assume all risks. Unless otherwise limited by law, the author will not be held responsible or liable in any way for the information within this book, and you agree to absolve the author of any liability or loss that you or any other person may incur from its information, including accidents, delays, injuries, harm, loss, damage, death, lost profits, personal or business interruptions, misapplication of information, physical or mental disease, condition or issue, or otherwise, and to absolve the author of any liability for any type of damages, including direct, indirect, special, incidental, equitable, or consequential loss or damages that may result from this book. You hereby fully and completely hold no harm against, indemnify, and release the author from any and all causes of action, allegations, suits, claims, damages, or demands whatsoever, in law or equity, that may arise in the past, present or future that are in any way related to this book.

CONTENTS

CONTENTS

Dedication

For Anew.

INTRODUCTION
Bipolar or Trans-Conscious?

"The greatest service I can do for someone is so they have an aha! moment or epiphany.[It] sets people on their own journey."

- Don Estes

Congratulations. You've won the lottery. The odds of being born are one in 400 trillion according to a Tedx talk by Mel Robbins. In mania, BOOM, justifiably you are ecstatic to be impossibly alive as a unique and wonderous human being. I wonder if you can resonate. Ten years ago, I received a diagnosis that changed my life: bipolar 1 with psychotic features. That was after my first two-month long mania that turned into psychosis. My journey has included six stays in psychiatric hospitals, two years living in supported housing, days when I've felt like I was dying, and days that I tried to kill myself. Bipolar disorder has taken many lives. Bipolar has added to my life. The bipolar diagnosis is part of why I'm alive today since it's connected me with resources and supports.

Despite the challenges I've faced living with bipolar 1, in parts of mania I've had positive and potential experiences. Bipolar has a mysterious allure. Bipolar mania is profound in that it can shine a light on what is hidden, making it more real than what we call reality. It illuminates beauty, ecstasy, trauma, pain, suffering, depression, and parallel realities—and more dimensions of our humanness than would otherwise be available. This only adds to its realness. It gives more energy, more information, new perceptions, and responses. Bipolar includes the whole spectrum of human experience from our best possible to our worse imaginable self. I'm not claiming a cure for bipolar disorder. This book is not meant to diagnose, prevent, or cure any disease. When I'm saying there's no cure for bipolar disorder, I'm also saying there is no cure for parallel realities, quantum physics, and the mysteries of the Universe. This is my attempt to make more of mania effable, so that it won't continue to "EFF" us up through its seeming ineffability. Glimpses into mania yielded a wealth of millions of words. The word "mania" is in these pages 717 times. That makes 718.

I am hoping to bring new meaning to the conversation about mania. I'm talking from "full-blown" mania associated with bipolar 1. We aren't talking about it; we are speaking from it and as it. There's a big difference. The intention is to lean into the so-called euphoric and ecstatic percentile of mania and aim to be a safe space for dialogue. The breadth of this slice of the overall bipolar experience and its tsunami of ideas is underrepresented and misrepresented through omission. On a questionnaire to score mania, the only euphoric traits they could identify were "looks happy and cheerful" and "verbalizes feelings of well-being."[i] The Manic Rating Scale shows and example of the small clinical scope available by looking 'objectively' at mania from the outside.[ii] The part of mania that leads us to clinical settings is not the whole story. Doctors tell us not to think about it too much, but I did it anyway. We will cover a vast matrix of mania and bipolar positives, nuances, and paradoxes from the inside out so anyone can connect to mania, even non-experiencers. By philosophizing our way into bipolar mania and psychosis, we may philosophize our way through it by engaging with it differently. Mania can be an opening—a revelatory element that our lives were deprived of.

THE TABOO

It's taboo to talk about the positive lived experiences of bipolar disorder. I saw on a reddit forum where people with a bipolar diagnosis were talking about how mentioning the positives in manic episodes is "dangerous," "insulting," "nonsense," "running wild," and "a terrible disservice to people's suffering." Yet, my work is to remove this taboo and speak about the positives. I don't want you to think I haven't struggled and suffered just like you. The last time I was in the psych ward was three years ago, and I nearly died in the process—again. I was stable with zero mania for over three years. Stability is the gold-standard goal we are told is important. I am exploring new dimensions of plasticity with new tools to add another modulator dial to my dashboard. I can channel or harness the perceptions of the eyes of mania when I'm 100% not manic, stable, and on medications. I've made it into a useful skill that I can call upon. I'm channeling mania without being manic. This book is a mirror for you to harvest and harness what is gifted through mania to you. Our brains have a built-in bias towards negativity, so finding the positives takes some effort at first—an intentional shift in mindset. I admit, this book itself is manic. Mania removes our negativity bias, and we will challenge the negativity bias towards mania. Contrasting other books to this one will provide a balanced view rather than looking for a balanced view in this one. Here you'll find how and why this missing conversation has been dismissed.

Carl Jung said, "Loneliness is not a lack of people around you, it's a lack of opportunity to say things that matter to you." By exploring the whole range of my bipolar experiences without resisting them, and extrapolating new meaning, I have found, or better yet, created, order in the chaos, certainty in the uncertainty, and love from the suffering. I see the possibility that our bipolar lives can change for the better. Imagine that my words are speaking to the positives in your bipolar experiences, whether hidden, subtle, divine, repressed, happy, awe-struck, or grandiose. I am speaking to those states and traits. We deny looking at these experiences when we have a preconceived notion that it's "bad." This conclusion is second hand, told to us by others. If you've understood all you can from mania, then please put down this book and ask me for a refund. If you're ready, let's soar into the heights of mania we are told are off limits. Maybe they hold the key to our unlimited nature. If you are willing to accept these experiences as part of your life rather than disowning and resisting them out of fear and frustration, I'm here with you through each word, sentence, and paragraph. By the end, we will have a new common ground to stand on—our co-drafted and co-crafted context of bipolar consciousness.

Making Sense for Ourselves

Bipolar disorder is called a brain illness, so we assume we are understanding when we refer to it that way too. We welcome a way to make sense of ourselves. We can go much deeper than that. It's not irresponsible to understand mania. On the contrary, it's our responsibility to endeavor to because we are the only ones who can do it directly. Keeping our brain fresh by using it afresh is mental health. Everything we get from others is indirect, abstract, and conceptual. Relying on medical paradigm language is a good Band-Aid, but a Band-Aid left on too long prevents full healing. We don't need to get angry at the Band-Aid, nor do we have to yell at bipolar people who wish to take the Band-Aid off, see what happens, and share their thoughts. We can learn from mania and build an understanding rather than live in fear.

In essence, we are talking about what is now called mental illness in terms that don't depend on or stem from the pathology narrative. Let's put it in positive terms here. We are spreading positive, growth oriented, and human potential ideas about mania, bipolar and even psychosis. We are closing the gap in consciousness between our regular consciousness and manic consciousness by building a bridge between the two with our own words, voice, and perception. We are planting seeds of manic consciousness in mainstream life.

I'm not saying that you should stop using the medical paradigm or go off your medications and be manic. Medications are an important piece of the puzzle—a chemical control stick for chaos in consciousness. They are vital for harvesting our mania by slowing down our brain so we can work to bring its wisdom into our daily life in manageable bits the brain can integrate. Harvesting the wisdom takes work, like bees work to gather honey. This book isn't 'antipsychiatry' and I'm not 'antipsychiatry.' I'm taking four medications while I write this. Psychiatry brought me back from the parallel world of mania and psychosis two handfuls of times. I'm grateful to psychiatry for being the portal and anchor to the material world.

Through the inpatient unit landing pad, I was introduced and incubated in the psychosocial Clubhouse model. I had the space I needed to re-discover and re-create myself alongside wonderful people, peers and workers, who emanated unconditional positive regard. I had a fairytale journey, because besides the fifteen-minute psychiatrist or clinician appointments, I was immersed in the caring Clubhouse. When I took training to become a Peer Support Worker, I was shocked out of my privileged state. I felt extreme empathic vicarious trauma from working within the medical "care" part of the system. The whole energy of it was wrong and I felt it just shouldn't be designed by the clinical gaze. Thankfully, the amount of wonderful people who work in mental health overcompensates for the destructive nature of some aspects of it. As a peer, I couldn't hold up a boundary and spiraled into a traumatic hospital experience of my own. So, like many of us, I am critical of psychiatry and some of its unnecessary evils, so I use my lived experience lens to critique it too and include my anger. In the scale of consciousness created by Dr. David R. Hawkins[2], anger is a bridge to pride, and pride a bridge to courage and willingness. Looking back, I wouldn't change my journey because I've explored dimensions that few get the opportunity to and lived through the system that brought me back to tell the tale. Perhaps without the psych system, you wouldn't have found this book and I'd never have written it. So, this is an evolution from it, not a thing that happens without it, by denying it, or transporting to a parallel reality. It's up to us to evolve beyond.

The Way Through is to Walk Between

We need to walk in both worlds—the subtle and physical. By walking between worlds, we can make the best of both. I'm pro-subjective meaning making as well as using medical tools to play by the rules of the social-physical world. But the medical system isn't helpful for the dimensions of mania we're looking at in this book. In mania, we live in a mysterious climate, so we need more words to demystify the unknown: premonitions, extrasensory perceptions, synchronicities, information influx, downloading, channeling, time travel, and parallel realities to name a few. Perhaps there are numerous types or classes of synchronicities? We could make distinctions by coining new words. Yet neologisms are on the list of clinical indicators for bipolar disorder and schizophrenia in the DSM-5 or *Diagnostic and Statistical Manual Volume 5*.[3] In our game, BipolarMania, neologisms are reframed as an essential tool to re-uncover the vast unmapped linguistic, physical, energetic, and informational territory of manic consciousness. Neologisms can be re-contextualized as part of the positive psychology of mania when we consider their function differently. In the book *Psychiatry Disrupted*, Bonnie Burstow says the following about language:[4]

> For example, any action that helps de-medicalize the language used about people who process differently than those deemed "normal," or live in alternative realities, or are in emotional

turmoil could be seen as an abolitionist change, for if enough of the language shifted over time, it would chip away at the impression that psychiatrists work so hard at maintaining–that such states or ways of being are "medical issues" and hence the proper domain of doctors.

So, then what is our approach? Re-gaming bipolar. The game is called BipolarMania. Adding 'mania' to the end of a word adds the connotation of excitement, fun, and adventure. BipolarMania is a game played to emphasize and explore the positive aspects of the journey through heightened states of consciousness. The aspect of BipolarMania that digs in to harvest past manias is called Re-Uncovery. What is Re-Uncovery? It's the intentional processes of uncovering the meaning in our manic and bipolar experiences, on our own terms and in our own terms. Re-Uncovery is a new movement to 'Re-Uncover' what we discovered and experienced during our mania. We discovered a cure to our deepest wound– our forgotten originality. We cover it up and forget about it when we call it 'bad', but it's still there. We can look to our memories, notebooks, photos, videos, audios, poems, or other artworks to harvest our manias. Not only can we uncover the potential in mania, but we can also expand on it by zooming out and extrapolating more meaning. We can fill in the gaps. The process can be intense. This book is intense, and it's meant to be intense. The intensity connects us to manic information without needing to be manic–so you know you are a unique miracle again.

Re-Uncovery

Re-Uncovery is explored in addition to participating in the Recovery Movement. I've participated in the Recovery process for the last ten years, and four years ago, I engaged my process of Re-Uncovery. Mania leaves a blueprint that we can reach to with our braincells when we are no longer manic. Then mania serves its purpose; we close the gap between the content and context of daily life and that of the manic state. Everyday life is more meaningful while episodes or iterations of mania are more understandable, easier to integrate, less scary, less intense, and we can keep up.

Re-Uncovery includes four aspects:

Harvest: Re-uncovering the content and context of manic consciousness after we've returned to the cis state. This includes experiences, special messages, art etc.

Harness: Looking at mania and its content and context through human potential and positive psychology lenses. We look retrospectively at mania after it's over, or 'meta-mania.'

Philosophize: Engaging manic content and context to extrapolate and expand upon it in retrospect and in daily life. We need a philosophy of bipolarism.

Practice-Embody: Re-iterate to the next level through action.

Though the process may seem pseudo-theoretical, conceptual, or abstract, we will see clues, signs, situations, and events that show its practicality in daily life. Life becomes what you wish, yet at the same time, a surprise. What is new is always surprising, and what is surprising is indeed always new. When you are no longer surprised by the magic and mystery of participatory life, mania will have served its purpose of expanding our conception of life. This is expansionist, not reductionist.

What is the approach to Re-Uncovery? It lies in the workings of the manic mind. Manic thinking is a combination of divergent, creative, holistic/nonlinear, abstract, and lateral thinking as well as other subtle and undefined types mania can elucidate. You can get the most out of the new ideas in this book by using a kaleidoscope of these thinking types. To solely rely on critical thinking, agreeing or disagreeing, and liking and disliking what's said is to miss the point. There is no point and there are a million points. We aren't discussing linear and binarily divided consciousness but are weaving many strings in all directions. The subheadings are meant to insert a pause for the braincells to take a breath, not to be perfect topic divisions. If a point is mentioned and seems incomplete at first, see it as a puzzle piece to be put back down, only to easily slot it into place when other pieces allow more of the picture to emerge. If something is puzzling, either skim over if need be and peruse past it, pause and ponder, or put it away for the day. Let the world of experience in your subconscious weave into these words while you rest and digest. When your mind makes a connection, your consciousness is involved in a creative act and your braincells flex their cytoskeletic muscles. Make no mistake, we are going to grow and strengthen our braincells by putting them through a workout. We are building our consciousness, not an argument or proof. We are staying curious, wondering, and expanding. I'm not trying to say my truths are universal truths; these are my insights from my experiences. I hope this book will spark you and your brain to learn how to learn from mania, without being manic or craving it. The traits and qualities of mania do not require mania, though that's how we become aware of them. Rather than ignoring them, as we explore, we can adapt. The brain is most fundamentally designed to learn and to ignore information is to starve it of the opportunity to do what it's meant to do.

Orientations of Consciousness

Bipolarism is an orientation in consciousness. Just as we have sexual orientations, we have consciousness orientations, or orientations in consciousness. To assume that we all see the world the same linear logical way, with the same rationality, and that we should do so is a hallucination. I call myself 'trans-conscious.' What do I mean by trans-conscious? I have access to mainstream and manic consciousness, and I transition between the two modes or orientations. Sometimes our consciousness shifts on the inside. We experience a different physical reality on the outside that doesn't match the reality we're conditioned to interpret through our programming, or birth reality. We are learning the art of the state of mania and being trans-conscious. Humans are creating new terminology to reflect how individuals feel on the inside, regardless of their apparent outside form, like declaring our pronouns. People declare how they like to be referred to in the third person. I don't think anyone wants to have their consciousness referred to as mentally ill. We also need more room to be different in consciousness, information processing, and how we manifest reality for ourselves. We need to take back authority over our existence and provide space for this conversation outside the disease model.

Maybe consciousness overall is bipolar, and it can manifest and express itself anywhere between the poles. Humans have parsed out a small part of it and called the rest disease. We need diversity of perceptions and experiences as part of the neurodiversity of consciousness. Just as biodiversity ensures the continuance of life on Earth, surely neurodiversity ensures the survival of humanity. The Hearing Voices Movement and Transgender Movements are examples of current human rights movements; we can follow in their footsteps. This is how we can shrink our perceived need for the disease model when we meet our higher needs. The mental illness system will not disappear and cease to be available to us, but our own narrative and way of seeing ourselves will be predominant in our consciousness. The mental illness narrative will be a smaller and subservient part to a larger whole of subjectively meaningful integrated consciousness. Through Re-Uncovery, we won't crave mania as an escape because we can access it all the time.

Being Content with Context

This book is meant to provide a lot of context and philosophy for you to decide what's useful to you, compare realizations, not feel alone, and have a loose framework or mesh of ideas in which to place your own. It's participatory and sparks your brain to restart your subjective sense-making. Just as no two experiences of mania are alike, there may be no two ways that philosophizing about mania in retrospect are alike. Please remember to read this book as a primer for your own insights, both re-uncovered and new. What's important in reading this is what is alchemized in you—what you see as a flash of insight. Read between the lines and fill the gaps with what your consciousness intimates to you. It doesn't matter if what I say is absolutely true—it's not. It was subjectively true in a snippet of space-time in my mindscape.

What's important is to re-spark your ability to do this for yourself. Otherwise, it's just recording other people's information and recalling memories. When you learn to learn for yourself again, and from yourself, you fulfill the earnest desire of the human brain. Then you don't need any book because you can read life directly in the moment. Life is a beautiful game, and beauty is in the eyes of you, the beholder. We create beauty when we see it. Think, process, and integrate this in the language that is meaningful to you. Maybe you coined a more suitable term than trans-conscious. Instead of having a few steppingstones across a river, we can fill it in and make bridges. Hopefully, this is a helpful guide for your own need to consider your experiences your own way. This provides context, not answers. That way you can create your own answers. By the time your finished reading this, you can write your book too. You don't even have to publish it.

Take a minute to think about your bipolar journey so far. What do you tell yourself? What have you been told to think about bipolarism? What's your story? And don't worry, you don't have to tell the world you're going to embark on a journey to explore bipolarism in a different way. This is for you. Otherwise, you may be accused of lacking insight into your illness, if you haven't been already. Or better yet, get your support team to read along with you. We all struggle with who society says we are and who we think we are. Just because we've been told we have a lifelong serious mental illness doesn't mean you can't create the life and become the person you want to and were meant to be. We can keep the illness identity as long as it serves us, and we can have other identities that crowd out thoughts of disorder. We've been imprinted with a strong, negative bias towards ourselves that sadly prevents us from trying or thinking that trying is even worth it. Diagnosis is helpful to reduce uncertainty, and medications can help reduce chaos and stress. But we can't use our diagnosis as an excuse to stop using our brains. Use it or lose it applies even more *because* we are on medications. We will focus on our assets rather than deficits and 'needs.' We are going to repossess our identity. We are moving towards higher intentions for mania to direct its surplus of energy consciously.

When we ask these questions of ourselves, we are in a dialogue with ourselves and the Universe. We draw information from the Universe. Mania is an information-philic state; we are drawn to information and draw information to us. We are infophiles and we need to mine for the meaning and significance. During my first mania, I channeled and downloaded a lot of information. It was hard to separate the signal from the noise to find and create the meaning. I've sorted and pruned thousands of hours' worth of information to filter the ideas down to what seems significant. It's only the tip of the iceberg, and I'm just one bipolar iceberg. How can we harvest and process the information? I created an information management process. It's called "Self-dialogue." We'll go into the details in chapter three. Self-dialogue is part of Re-Uncovery, though not all of it. We will be able to deal with information overload rather than ignore it. Through Self-dialogue, I create insight into my subjective and living experience of trans-conscious phenomenon. This self-understood information is important. We can build a foundation—a mountain of meaning and significance—to bathe in.

Reverse-Inclusion to Synchronicity

In mania, we clearly see that reality can and does work in mysterious ways. Medications help us to forget what we experienced and move on, but it's only suppressed. Our manic states of mind are meaningful states. Our ways of being are meaningful. The mental illness system tells us it's all meaningless. The mental health system discourages us from philosophizing about our experiences. They indicate that to do so could make our illness worse because we are humoring delusions. We are told to forget our direct experiences and believe instead that we are crazy. Here, we are calling forth a "meaning model" of mania, Trans-Consciousness, and other alternative realities. What's great about a meaning model is that it matters how the experiencer sees it, feels it, and lives it. What we say is primary and takes precedence. Also, we can make up and fabricate as many meanings and interpretations as we like.

We can live by synchronicity and let what's meaningful in our hearts be our guide. And because we've experienced mania, we have a key to access new information and meaning like few others on Earth do. We also tap into the magic of the source code—the malleability and creative nature of language. We originate ideas, we don't think of them in the traditional or classical sense. They arise from the origin, now. We see differently. You could say we are 'Manian,' almost like it's a new religion, and we exist in every culture. We are borderless and colorless. Now is the time to stop being faceless and voiceless.

A mental illness diagnosis can make us feel and experience exclusion from society. We are called outsiders. We want to be included. This book is also about inclusion in a totally different way.

An episode of bipolar mania can lead us to being hospitalized in a psych ward and treated with medications, isolation, or electric shock. Our rights and freedoms are taken away in many instances. As part of the recovery movement, the mental health system puts tireless effort into bringing us back to consensus reality in hopes that we can one day be full citizens in society again.

A couple decades ago, there was little belief that people could recover from serious mental illnesses. We were institutionalized and excluded from the community–given ice baths, insulin comas, and lobotomies. While I wouldn't wish any of this on anyone, there are many aspects of bipolar mania that I wish everyone could experience. I'd imbue it in a little glass stone and hand it over during a synchronistic conversation and seal the deal with a 30-second eye gaze without blinking. A gift for the so-called normal people who've never experienced mania is access to all the benefits of mania without having to be manic.

If you don't know what it's like to be manic, imagine all the obvious and subtle forms of inner and outer oppression impinging on your circumstances and psyche suddenly being removed without cause. You feel lighter and in awe of everything because it's been made new. In mania, it happens for real. We are all living in a world that oppresses the human spirit in one form or another, and we may not even know since we can't see beyond it. It makes sense to work to include non-experiencers in the world of mania because in simplest terms, it's a prolonged temporary relief from programmed oppression we all are infected with. With this we are on common ground. We all have an oppressed and an unoppressed version of ourselves, and we can unlock our mind-body by connecting them together in an instant. This is the light switch in mania.

Beyond being distracted by programmed oppression, the world is mysterious, unknown, and magical. When we see life as it is, we appear to be manic relative to the masses who are still oppressed. This makes a lot more sense than calling people who can see beyond the veil mentally ill. We aren't better or worse than anybody else for the temporary loss of oppression. We haven't yet been able to include others in lifting the veil as much as others try to re-include us in putting it back over our eyes. Rather than miss who we were and try to get us to recover into the capitalistic patriarchy, maybe you'll see the world you are missing out on, so we all have a higher chance of discovering it. We've paid a big price, but there is more to life than what we've been sold through our upbringing. I don't draw conclusions, but I paint from disillusionment because I've seen a different world. This isn't logical but it's not illogical either. When more see the truth, it will be assimilated into logic and called logical because we'll have the language to verbalize it. Not all that is logical need arise through science and objectification. At the same time, what we experience is explained in the science, but we need re-uncovery to extrapolate it ourselves from within the lived experience lens.

With this declared, we are giving ourselves permission to include ourselves in the human potential movement, and normal people in the re-uncovery of the uncaused crazy joy of being human. And we must keep re-uncovering it, just like advertisers will play the same commercial twice in a three-minute block. But as a YouTube video about Neitchze by Academy of Ideas said, "Why should anyone pay attention to ideas on how to 'become who you are' from a man who went mad?"[5] Because we want to share the fruits of harvesting our mania. I'm glad there are so many quotes to draw on to lend light to these possibilities.

Permission to Come Out as Trans-Consciousness?

I've shared my recovery story and my journey of being a mental patient on many occasions over the years in hopes that I might help people have an easier time or family members have hope and compassion for their loved one. Let's drop the concept of help in favor of empowering your own mind to create context and to self-direct your own understanding. You are who and what's important, not the words in these pages. I'm excited to articulate my bipolar trans-conscious journey on and in my own terms. I've realized it's not so much a journey but an exploration, since my consciousness is not linear. My sharing is a coming out, not via a recovery story of a mental patient, but as a trans-conscious philosopher and explorer. Many symptoms of mental illness are also signs of human potential, breakdown, the dark night of the soul, spiritual emergency, breakthrough, awakening, and transformation. My wish is to inspire you to have faith in your own eyes, ears, body, brain, intelligence, insights, and more, so we can talk to ourselves and each other on a whole new level. We need to talk ourselves out of being programmed with self-stigma, and we need to talk ourselves into our dreams and the unique roles we can step into in our life and in culture. If we break the taboo, it can abolish the concept of stigma.

I love my manic mind, with all its dimensions, depths, heights, and aspects. In mania, I saw the world is made of love and interconnectivity and I resonate with the word Gaia—the vast organism that is the Earth. I love my bipolar intelligence because I can sense the Gaian mind. It makes consciousness into a living work of art so that I can channel gifts, special powers, talents, and secrets. The false disengages and the truth of the power of being a human being takes place. When I see mania from a human potential and positive psychology lens, the game of life is fun. I love reframing and extrapolating from the fluid and fluxing manic vantage points.

We are giving ourselves permission to decide and create what our experiences mean. If you've experienced mania, then you've had a 'glimpse.' A glimpse of what? You decide. We need to speak of our human potential. Human potential and mental illness are overlapping concepts and realities. Bipolar people and other labelled consciousness will give themselves permission to speak the human potential they discovered in themselves in non-ordinary states of consciousness.

I have so much to share with you and you're not alone. This is my message, not peer to peer, but manic to manic. I wish you find a friendly stranger in these pages in your quest for meaning in your experiences and the creation of your dreams. I will share personal stories and examples, insights, hypotheses, extrapolations, ideas, and musings. I may be called crazy, ill, lacking insight into my disorder, grandiose, delusional, hallucinating—but then I'm no worse off than the paradigm from which I started. I will speak freely to participate in creating diversity in consciousness. It's time to inspire, celebrate, and amplify bipolarism in new ways. As cliché as it is, if this book inspires just one person, it was worth it. I wish you to find something profound in these pages.

Here are some ideas of what you might get out of this game:

- Develop your expertise on yourself.

- Fuel and nourish your trans-conscious brain.

- Remember many thoughts and perspectives you had in mania.

- See that mania is a natural process that is regarded and handled unnaturally.

- Stop being shamed by and apologizing for the experiences.

- Understand the ego is like an electric fence that keeps us limited.

- Be in awe of bipolar and the strength it takes to live it.

- Harness the Power of Now and relate it to bipolarism.

- Retrain and readjust your eyes to see the impossible again in daily life.

- Have enough meanings to create a manic context and philosophy.

- Enough manic philosophers can create a movement of re-uncovery.

- See manic energy as our birthright. As children, we have this energy, and then we are trained out of it. It's not something inhumane or foreign but forgotten.

- Lean towards 'abilitation' and re-uncovery of manic traits and recovery of old capacities.

- See that we face common challenges living the experience at different stages.

- Feel safer in your experience and toward your future experience by making sense of your experiences yourself. Rest in your own understanding and ability to understand now and always.

- Notice two different ways of being, manic and normal, correlate with two totally different worlds.

- Begin to make paternalism and oppression in the system obsolete by moving towards self-direction, self-discovery, meta-mania, and re-uncovery.

- Think about your own bipolar praxis or "customs" to design a custom life.

- Acknowledge how mania affects our sensitivity and change in views and values.

- Think of this process as a game because games are fun.

- Learn by epiphany.

- Get your power back.

- Move from fearful to fascinated.

- Use this book to have a dialogue with yourself and write your own book.

- Break the taboo of talking and thinking in positive terms about mania, at least with yourself, me, and a community of us.

- Start to make all your favorite grandiose delusions for the best of humanity come true.

- Get re-excited about your dreams.

DISCLAIMER – EXCLAIMER

"Nobody benefits from dire predictions."

- Mary Ellen Copeland

Before we talk about Re-uncovery, we need to acknowledge the incredible suffering involved in bipolar. If you are in crisis, now is not the time to read this. Find your relevant crisis outreach information or hotline and go from there. On July 16, 2022, in the USA, "988" will be the new three-digit dialing code that will go to the National Suicide Prevention Lifeline. Each country is unique and it's up to you to know the resources to save your life before you fall into a crisis. When in doubt, call 911, or the emergency line of your country. Your will to live is imprinted and planned in the moments where crisis is absent. Falling from the heights of mania, surviving psychosis, and managing depression is scary, harsh, painful, torturous, unforgiving, and sometimes unrelenting. There are many times I've endured physical and mental agony, unable to move, begging for mercy and grace. The National Institute of Mental Health says bipolar disorder is a "mental disorder that causes unusual shifts in mood, energy, activity levels, concentration, and the ability to carry out day-to-day tasks."[6] An estimated 4-19% of people with bipolar disorder end their life.[7] The DSM-5, states that people diagnosed with bipolar disorder are 15 times more likely than the general population to die by suicide and amount to one quarter of all suicides.[3] "Serious and persistent mental illness" can decrease a person's lifespan between 11-30 years, especially if substance use and lifestyle factors are involved.[8]

Bipolar not only impacts life expectancy, but it can also seriously diminish quality of life. The side effects of medications can lead to weight gain, metabolic syndrome, diabetes, tardive dyskinesia, and a mountain of other problems.[9] Psychiatric medications don't work for everyone or can stop working.[10] Here, in serious cases, people go to "refractory treatment." Rather than putting the blame on the individual for being treatment-resistant and throwing in the towel, we need more choices and treatment options.

The system focuses on what they call positive and negative symptoms of bipolar disorder. The positive symptoms are undesirable added symptoms and not actually something positive. Positive symptoms include hearing voices, delusions, and believing they have special powers. Negative symptoms include reduced motivation, monotone speech, inexpressiveness, and a lack of spontaneity. Regarding bipolar disorder, the word 'positive' has already been coopted as a detrimental symptom. I'm not alone when I say that bipolar has many positive 'positive symptoms' and they are added gifts. Not only that, some so-called negative symptoms of bipolar disorder also have hidden positive aspects that are nearly impossible to see by the outside observer. Bipolar temporarily deactivates our default-mode false-self. We were programmed that way; it's not our natural state. We get to live in and try on alternative modes of being and experiencing life in mania. Even though we are tasked with recouping our past mode of daily life functioning in recovery, we now know something else is possible—and we can't forget. The ripples of mania remain as a blueprint in our hearts. Our hearts yearn to get back to the manic way of being. Mania can trick us into thinking we don't need our body or Earth for our mission. And that is a catastrophic mistake.

Bipolar is serious and persistent, and we must persistently take our safety seriously. Bipolar can trick us into leaving our bodies and our loved ones. Having a plan to stay safe when things get out of control is essential. Where I'm from, before leaving the hospital, a clinician creates a safety plan in case of a relapse into crisis. A safety plan, crisis plan, advance directive, Ulysses agreement, or Wellness Recovery Action Plan (WRAP) is a vital pre-thought-out action. I have a WRAP plan and I'm a facilitator. You can get the WRAP app in the app store for free and fill in the sections or look for a local group in your area. Crisis line phone numbers can be kept handy in a favorites list in your contacts. Later in the book, there is a section on creative safety. Feel free to skip to it and read it if you don't feel completely safe and trusting of yourself no matter the scenario. Keep in mind, my ideas are not a formula. What feels creatively safe for me might make you feel worse. The safer we feel, the less fear interferes with or distorts our exploration. We want to make positive and rich aspects of bipolar perceptible while putting the old paradigm in perspective from 30,000 feet. We can look from 30,000 feet, but never jump. Having a plan to keep ourselves safe helps pre-practice what to do when we don't feel safe or enter a crisis. When you are in, or anywhere near crisis, that isn't the time to explore the upper echelon of a manic's hierarchy of needs.

Get help, even if it seems like it's doing more harm than good. You can make it through. I captured this quote from a TV show featuring a man who later ended his life. He said, "I didn't want to go to the hospital and start from square zero." Yes, the psych ward is square zero. I've felt this too. Truly, we can start from square zero. We do start from square zero. With bipolar, learning to start again from square zero is a must. It's part of the process. Because it's cyclical, we must start from square zero, like we did the first time. And we can get better at it. We're like cats. We have 9 lives. Go to the psych ward in peace and don't let the fear, anger, hate, or violence win. It's not the end. It's another beginning. I've survived multiple excruciating, torturous, agitated suicidal states that I didn't think I could take for a millisecond longer. Freeze and don't fight or flee. The evil tries to trick us into reacting. When we don't react, evil has no vehicle or fuel. The mercy of compassion and grace is real. Please stay here for the ones you love, who love you, who've loved you, who you are yet to love, and who are yet to love you. You have no idea how important you are. The world needs you. Dr. Peter Breggin said in his book Toxic Psychiatry, "Ultimately, every individual must choose whether or not to overcome any hardship or oppression inflicted by the family, society, or psychiatry. Human beings retain a measure of free will as long as they remain conscious."

Again, this book is not meant to diagnose, prevent, or cure any disease. Please don't take anything in this book as medical advice or reason to delay seeking medical attention or treatment from qualified mental health professionals. They want to help, and they are the only ones officially trained to help. Let them help, and they will. I'm sending appreciation to the professionals who've helped in the best way they knew how. This book is only for potential, possible, experimental, pragmatic, entertainment, magic, mysterious, lived-experience, educational, dialogical, and re-uncovery purposes. You should only explore these higher needs of bipolar when basic needs and recovery goals have been met. Also, I'd like to put out a trigger alert as I do share stories and information that could be triggering. I hope that most of what I share aren't triggers but "sparkers" that ignite and unfold the magic of energy, information, and meaning. I hope we can start to say "me too" in a positive way regarding bipolar and contribute to the work of all the peers of yesterday, today, and tomorrow.

I want to acknowledge the incredible and infinite diversity of bipolar experience. My intention is not to paint my experience and ideas as typical, correct, or of any more or less value than anyone else's. I only truly know my experience, so I have no idea—nor claim to know—what pertains to anyone else. What's helpful to some could be harmful to others. You must decide what's beneficial and healthy for you. This is part of developing and tuning our ability to create our bipolar senses. I'd like to thank all the peers and advocates who have shared their work so I could find it. And for being crazy enough to change the world. Game on.

HOW TO USE THIS LIVING THE EXPERIENCING BASED BOOK

"Reading is like a software update for your brain."

- James Clear

We are going on a journey to make sense and meaning out of bipolar states that we've been told:

- make no sense

- have no meaning

- have no function or purpose

- are only detrimental

- are delusions and/or hallucinations

- are symptoms of our disease or illness

- are lacking insight into our illness

- will make us worse if we try to make sense of them

- and whatever else diverts our attention from what we think independently

All the above talking points and more are deeply ingrained in our minds after our post-diagnosis education. We need a fresh start. The following principles are shared here from the Hearing Voices Network[11] to quickly erase the old mindset and adopt a new one. They're grounded in 35 years and thousands of people with lived and living experience of voices, visions, and extraordinary experiences. We can draw on their strength to feed our own and give ourselves permission to speak about our experiences on our own terms, despite how we've been educated.

- *We are free to interpret our experiences however we choose*

- *We are free to challenge social norms*

- *We are free to talk about anything*

- *We are free to change our minds at any time*

In alignment with these principles, I declare my freedom to interpret my experiences however I choose, challenge social norms regarding acceptable perspectives of bipolar, talk about anything, and change my mind at any time. Some of my chosen and self-created methods include creative perception and extrapolation, neologisms, re-languaging, lateral thinking, divergent thinking, meta-mania, and insight into my experiences. To extrapolate means to "project, extend, or expand (known data or experience) into an area not known or experienced so as to arrive at a usually conjectural knowledge of the unknown area."[12]

Meta-mania is a kind of 'retrospecting' and it's part of Re-Uncovery. Meta-mania uses extrapolative thinking to reflect on past manias to connect the dots for a clearer bigger picture. Our mind, brain, and consciousness are fulfilled in its purpose each moment it discovers something new or makes sense of something for itself. Since perception is participatory and creative, when we participate in creating our perceptions, life, nature, and the Universe are fulfilled through us. The power of our own consciousness to create is fulfilling. In this state, life is more an active, inside-out process than a passive, outside-in one. In the first we have creative power, in the second, we give our power away.

Personal meaning is golden—it's a compass. Otherwise, we are living someone else's life, or a life laid out for us. In a video by the Hearing Voices Network, they talked about their studies on individuals who attended Hearing Voices groups to see why they were so effective and "one factor that seems especially important is that they allow each person to make sense of their experiences using a framework that fits their individual circumstances."[11] By creating your own framework, you have the best chance to craft one that fits you.

When we were kids, we insisted on figuring things out for ourselves. We would protest if our parents tried to show us how to do something. The natural urge to grow and learn is slowly programmed out of us. We don't notice, just like a frog in a pot of water doesn't notice the change of temperature if it's slow enough. Rather than jumping out of the open pot to freedom, it boils. We learn the answers come from books, TV, and the internet formulated by someone else who happens to know better than us. School is mostly memorization and regurgitation through tests or raising our hand to get the right answer. We form an ego or false-self that lives our lives for us as a protection mechanism against these disembodied, nonsensical methods called learning. In mania, we jump out of the pot of the society that tried to boil us. Life feels new, rich, and meaningful. We see everything afresh because we are looking with fresh eyes. We absorb new ideas like sponges and access information we never thought of before. It feels like we are channeling or downloading information from another frequency or dimension.

How can you participate fully with this book? If you read something that resonates, a powerful way to engage deeper is to write this insight out by hand, look at it while relaxing your eyes and say it out loud. This is a kind of hand-eye-voice coordination. Writing by hand initiates a co-creative co-authorship that starts the process of building a network of bipolar meaning. By relaxing our eyes, we allow the information to get past our focal vision, or limits of the ego, and into the wholistic vision in the brain, which in turn creates a resonance that can lead to your insights. Speaking it out loud initiates the sound vibrations that bring us together to create a new paradigm, no matter where we are in the world. Through us, the Universe can sense a tangible signal and respond with feedback if it aligns with the new paradigm. A major part of the new paradigm is direct communication with the Universe. Through oneness, the Universe in relationship with us, as Gaia and nature, can materially unfold what we create subtly. The Universe can build insights into the material world, as more people consider them and resonate with them. First, there was the word, and we have this creative power and much more. Often, we try and go around and tell people about all the magic we see, and we only get thrown away. We can also spell it out to each other, from afar, and create the same possibilities. We can change the fabric of consciousness.

If the hand-eye-voice coordination strategy isn't interesting to you, I encourage you to at least write out your findings and 'aha's' that arise in your consciousness. Look at what you wrote with relaxed eyes, then say them out loud. You could voice them right away or save them until you've explored the meta-mania section in chapter 3. Additionally, if you have a bunch of writing you did in previous iterations of mania, on paper or in a computer somewhere, that is part of your "harvest." Your harvest is important for your journey and the evolution of consciousness and culture. Hold onto your harvest as you may be able to save the seeds and plant them when the time comes.

Framing common language among experiencers, language we coin and create, is one of our gifts. Re-uncovering and reflecting on our subjective participatory perceptions can crowd out the memes and programming of psychiatry to an appropriate portion of our life. We can overwrite what we were told with the integrations and extrapolations of our original, firsthand perceptions. We can create our own 'heard' immunity to what others have said we should think about ourselves. "Insight into your illness" can become "insights from your stillness" and "chemical imbalance" can become "alchemical balance." We must create what we want to see and hear to take the place of carefully crafted medical jargon and talking points. Only we can do this. Let's stop being marginalized with the assumptions from others that it's all nonsense. There is meaning in what's called "madness." This goes for all of us. Physicist Dr. David Bohm said, "It's very important that it happens together. If one individual changes, it will have very little general effect. But if it happens collectively, it means a lot more. If some of us come to the 'truth,' while a lot of people are left out, it's not going to solve the problem."[13] One person who harvests, practices, and embodies mania has way less power than two, ten, a hundred, or a thousand. If we each did so separately, that's amazing. Once as a group we start to communicate as we choose, it could be exponential.

To make it easier to participate, here is a quick "Harvest Your Mania" Template with some ideas for categories for your thoughts as you go along. It's to capture whatever you recall from your experiences as you read this as well as whatever new comes to mind. You can jot it in a journal or in your inotes. Feel free to create your own categories. In chapter 3, we'll get into a deeper process and the template will come in handy.

Information:

- Insights:
- Innovations:

- Ideas:
- Synchronicity and Quantum Weirdness:
- Quote from Book:

Capacities:

- Mission:
- Passions/Interests/Values:
- Notes to Self:
- Crisis Notes:
- New Traits, Skills, Gifts and Talents:
- Delusions and Dreams to Come True:

Creativity:

- Comedy/Song Lyrics:
- Poetry, Song Lyrics, and Titles:
- Neologisms Lexicon:

Practical Dashboard:

- To Do Today:
- Time Sensitive:
- Creative To Do List:
- Acts of Kindness and Altruism:
- Shopping List:
- Family Related Tasks:
- Maintenance:
- Tasks:
- Gigs/Services/Business:

Learning:

- Read:

- Research:

- Food and Nutrition:

- Alternative Mental Health Study:

- Projects:

- Micro Projects:

- Me Only Projects:

- Delegate/Outsource:

- Project Help:

- Sharing:

Whether you've been at this for years or you're newly diagnosed, by facing and engaging with your experiences through re-uncovery and meta-mania, you can restore trust in your perceptions. We can co-create our possible self and our dream world. We can transform from fate to destiny. We need to think and see differently, super-imposing human potential and positive psychology onto mania, and expanding the definition of what it means to be human. The game is as small or as large as we want to make it. The first part of the game is to break the taboo and amplify speaking on our own terms about manic consciousness, first to ourselves, the Universe, each other, friendly strangers, and then people we know. Usually, we start with people we know, then psychiatrists. Don't talk about 'light' club. To keep up to date with the evolution of everything Bipolar Game Changer visit:

https://linktr.ee/bipolargamechanger

Part
ONE

Away from the
Past Meaningless Mental Illness

"But I say: go beyond the impossible, see what happens!"
- J. Krishnamurti

Chapter 1

BUILDING A FOUNDATION OF MANIC MEANING

A BIPOLAR TRAIN RIDE TO THE WORLD OF MANIA

*"You have to do whatever it is you
can't not do."*

- Luisa Rey, in the movie Cloud Atlas

The first time I heard the term "bipolar disorder" I was in a training to be an inline skating instructor. Years later in 2011, I heard it again for the second time. That January, I was on a thirty-two-hour train ride to California. When the train stopped at Portland Station, a man in his late 50's entered the train and plopped down his stuff on a seat in the row in front of me. Somehow, a small exchange ensued, after which he looked at me, pondering with his head tilted sideways, before picking up his stuff and switching to the seat beside me. He was headed to Los Angeles. He kindly shared lively conversation as well as the fruits and veggies he'd meticulously packed for the long journey. We shared hours of conversation before strategizing that he should sleep on the seats while I curl up on the floor for maximum comfort for both of us. On the way to my stop in Santa Barbara, I started getting nervous about the hostel. I'd never traveled by myself before and I was a bit of a chicken. He offered to drive me back to Santa Barbara from LA if I got off the train with him.

As we neared Santa Barbara station, his disposition changed. He seemed irritated, and shared he had bipolar disorder and was on medication for it. He said he had been on an online poker winning streak. His family took the winnings he'd withdrawn and made him stop playing. He had promised to take the medications for his family's sake, even though it took the 'magical luck' away from him. Unbeknownst to him, he did help me get to my destination. After listening to his story, I was less afraid to get off the train than to stay on it. I didn't really know what bipolar disorder was, but I found myself wondering who I'd been sitting with all that time. It was an easy decision to detrain at my stop.

In retrospect, it feels like a foreshadowing moment. The six weeks I stayed in Santa Barbara were full of wonder, mystery, and synchronicity—some kind of magic luck. When I returned home, I didn't think the magic and synchronicity would have any new fuel to keep going. To my surprise, they continued for a month. I kept following the signs and slept two hours a night. Then it flipped into a month-long psychosis. The four-month process felt rich and spiritual and terrifying. I didn't know if I was becoming enlightened or going crazy. I ended up in a psych ward, sitting in front of a psychologist telling me I had bipolar 1 disorder with psychotic features. That was the third time I heard about bipolar disorder, and they were talking about me. Since then, whether 'I am bipolar' or 'I have bipolar,' bipolar has had me and it hasn't let me go. To summarize, I've been hospitalized six times totaling several months and have been on a dozen different medications. I've had long stints of depression and numerous super energetic manias followed by psychosis. A bipolar 1 disorder diagnosis means I have, and will likely always have, this so-called severe and persistent mental illness. Psychotic features tagged on the end is a bonus; it means it's the most severe form. And I count myself lucky.

When I was first read my diagnosis, my first thought was "that's not it." I didn't say as much at the time because I was cornered in a room by a doctor in a building backed by hundreds of years of psychiatric tradition. The four months of extraordinary experiences that led to my diagnosis, and any since mean infinitely more than a short scientific phrase could ever encapsulate. When I heard bipolar disorder, I knew it was designed to discourage sharing any subjectively perceived significance. Anything I did share would be seen as a symptom by the psychiatric framework. They were clear that I was ill, and they were there to put a stop to it at a high cost to my identity, physical health, longevity, and life in my years.

A few years went by before I saw signs to look back at my experiences in a meaningful way. I could never forget their significance, even while thoroughly engaged in the recovery process. Since 2014, I've been crazy about making meaning and insights out of mania and psychosis. Paradoxically, by doing this, psychiatry would say I lack insight into my illness. The "insight into my illness" talking point is a catch-22 because if we think we're not ill, it's proof of our illness. To think of bipolar in terms other than illness, we must lack insight into our illness. We need to remember there is more to the bipolar experience than illness. Indeed, we aren't trying to have insight into our illness, we are creating wisdom. There is more to life than illness, even a bipolar life. The benefit of lacking insight into our illness is that we can create and harvest insights into the unknown, uncertain, chaotic, and synchronous. I came up with my own philosophy because the medical ideology is limited in what it has to offer. I listened to myself, Gaia, and the Universe and discovered my bipolar has meaning.

MANIA, MEANING, AND MEANINGLESSNESS

"Nothing interesting begins with knowing,
it begins with not knowing."

 - Beau Lotto, Neuroscientist

A Game to Get the Meaning from Special Messages

As human beings, we have the capacity for new meaning. I'm not talking about looking up a new word in the dictionary to learn its meaning. We can conceive, alchemize, and birth new meaning through us. Research points out living with the treatments and socioeconomic factors that come with a diagnosis shortens our life span.[47] However, our meaning span, or the depth, breadth, and height of the meaning we can access in our life is exponential. If we access it, time will be filled with riches and seem to pass more slowly, whether we live longer or not. I want to let you in on the secret of how to create new meaning. Start from not knowing, just like the neuroscientist Beau Lotto points out in the quote above. I agree. We can 'know' and understand nearly anything when we know nothing. How? I don't know! It's the truth. Isn't that simple? Yet our default state is full of knowledge and memories chattering away. Knowing nothing is the hardest thing. Just try to silence your mind. And we don't know, we 'knew' because what we know is stored as memory. We see what we know when the mind chatters and wanders. We don't see what is new. What is, is new. When we stop projecting what we know, we can apprehend something outside of the known. The world is kind of magical and a bit mysterious. We can ask "What's new?" and wait for a surprise.

Living happens only when we are *in* the moment. When our mind wanders, we miss the moment. When we see the moment, life speaks to us, with us, through us, and as us. And life speaks and whispers the meaning of that moment in our consciousness, which we may or may not verbalize out loud. In mania, we speak it all out, logorrhea style. What we look at and give our attention to speaks to us and through us, plus the old thought commentary. We can commune and communicate with almost anything, except the people we know. Therefore, mania often initiates a deep connection with nature, animals, and strangers. In mania, a type of synesthesia happens. According to healthline.com, "synesthesia is a neurological condition in which information meant to stimulate one of your senses stimulates several of your senses."[14] We can hear what we look at and what we see. What we look at creates word-forms in our mind, and we can speak the words out loud or not. What we focus our attention on gives us information and speaks directly to us—it gives us what feels like special messages. The past chatter and commentary are old and not sensed as new or 'special.' New catalyzes intrinsically motivated learning.

Absurd Is the Word

How do we approach the novel game of deriving new meaning from the special messages of mania? It's neither meant to be a debate where the goal is to be right nor is it a discussion to facilitate an agreement. Dialogue, however, is about unfolding and sharing meaning, the approach we need for BipolarMania. Dialogue requires no consensus or hierarchy. Fluid understanding replaces fighting over fixed facts. Dialogue is more like weaving. No part of the weave is superior to the other, and the strings work together to create a greater whole. We will weave words into a type of framework or scaffolding that can support the unfolding of our lives touched by mania. We will intertwine the wisdom we re-uncover from manic consciousness with human potential and positive frames.

These words about mania, though painted through dialogue, are not the experience of mania itself. Alfred Korzybski said, "the map is not the territory"[15] and J. Krishnamurti said, "the word is not the thing."[16] The word 'mania' is like part of a 'map' and is not the vast lived experience, which is like the 'territory' of mania. In psychiatry, the concept of mania and its qualities are an abstraction or model based on clinical observations of our reports and behavior in the psych ward and not actual daily experiences. Clinical observations are from the outside and thought to be objective. In contrast, lived experiences are from the inside, and largely subjective. The diagnosis is made up of a bunch of words that make up the clinical 'map.' However, these descriptions still aren't the territory of mania. They can't resemble the territory as much as our own descriptions to ourselves from direct experience. Action in the territory of mania happens in a person experiencing the state of manic consciousness, and most of this happens outside the psych ward. Manic consciousness gives us access mania's parallel world or 'territory.' Though we can sometimes enthusiastically express ourselves in mania, unfortunately, we have been unsuccessful at communicating the territory of mania so far. Expression and communication aren't the same thing.

The clinical map may be helpful when we're in contact with clinicians. Speaking their language can assist them in better understanding so they may help us in the best way they can. The medical model can look at people in mania, but they still can't see and experience the territory like the person in mania can. We may seem confused by the end of an iteration of mania, and the medical system is equally oblivious when they think their maps correspond to the actual territory of mania. The medical model is not interested in the territory of mania. It's interested in blocking entry. They narrow their investigation down to our brain, but our brain is decoding and presenting a different world. Mania isn't in our brain. It's a territory, a reality, and our brains tune in to that level of consciousness and decode it via using new combinations of neural networks. Our brain is interpreting a different reality. The cause isn't the brain. Clinicians can't see our world, so they can only blame our brain. Our manic world is just as real. Let's not confuse the medical model map of mania and bipolar with the territory or consciousness of it to be the same as living experience.

The Crisis of Meaninglessness

The biggest crisis in the world is the sense of meaninglessness. It's not that life has no meaning. Meaning is everywhere; we just can't see it, interface with it, or engage with it because we live in a box. When we perceive new information, we have the opportunity to see or create new meaning. When the mind chatters on, it repeats, and we miss the ever-present opportunity to see the moment anew. Life is sensed as meaningless when we can't sense anything new. Every moment is new. We can't see that, and that's the biggest danger. Repetition has a high probability of being sensed as meaningless because it conveys no new information. We miss the profound in the subtle and the possibility of new meaning. New meaning doesn't have to be anything big, though it can be. The mind, brain, and consciousness are fulfilled when we notice something anew. The energy in mania allows us to see beyond the reality that the chatter of thought projects as our life.

Mania is beyond regular waking consciousness made by old thought. It's a super-awake state—we don't even need as much sleep. Seeing everything through new eyes, as new, creates energy. This is how fresh information enters the world. What we typically experience as waking consciousness doesn't give us much new information at all. In a normal waking state, we mostly live in our thought abstractions. As A Course in Miracles says, "my meaningless thoughts are showing me a meaningless world."[17] We don't have a relationship with the present moment. We have a relationship with our conflicting and distracting thoughts. One thought fights with another thought. When thoughts are at war with each other, the process that thought is meant for is being wasted. If you've ever driven home only to realize that you don't know how you got there, that's how we live most of the time. We need the thought abstractions to chatter on so that the body can be on autopilot. 95% of the time, we are on autopilot in a string of habits. We don't realize we're not present—the car is moving, but there is no driver. If we can maneuver a vehicle and be absent and unaware of our surroundings, we can do anything in that state. We aren't embodied and interfacing with what is happening. We aren't actual beings. When we are inattentive, there is a high cost to the Universe. We are living here without being in touch with the real world. We take the world's resources without being embodied to create with our consciousness. And I'm talking about the state of waking consciousness called normal.

So, is it just an illness or can we map unrealized possibilities and potential? Maybe it's both. Maybe one is our fate, and the other is our destiny? Maybe it doesn't matter. What does matter is that we need to challenge the belief that others know better about our experiences than us. We need to activate our brains like they were activated in mania—and what better way then by exploring the content and context of mania extrapolated creatively to other frames.

Overwritten Overlap of Human Potential

My work and play are to contribute to the literature of mania and bipolar that overlap with human potential and possibilities by looking at our lived and living experience. I'm learning from the context I've created with myself preventing cognitive decline, worsening of relapses, several hospitalizations, and the fear of living. I'm pursuing my dreams—and dreams make life worth living. Whether you've had a glimpse of mania or not, our exploration may be subtle, tacit, meaningful, and intangible, yet they affect our lives in tangible ways.

Positive psychology focuses on sources of psychological health, not deficiencies and pathology.[18] Why can't we have positive bipolarity and focus on the positives? Mania is a meaningful state of consciousness with a purpose—like fear, anger, and sadness—just at the other end of the emotional spectrum. If you've experienced mania like me, maybe you've tasted that magic and mystery—or drowned in it. Maybe you haven't had mania, but you have a loved one who has, and you're wondering what it could be like. Maybe you'd like to have the opportunity to absorb some manic memes and benefits without ever needing to enter mania. I mean, who doesn't want to be ridiculously, ecstatically happy for no reason and every reason—where you need nothing to be happy, but everything makes you happy? Maybe that's idealistic, even for some who has experienced mania. It may not be long before mania happens to you again. Maybe someone you know will be newly diagnosed. Mania doesn't discriminate. It's best to be prepared. Mania is a side effect of some medications. Mania seems like a sudden occurrence, but like a volcano that lays dormant, something is happening underneath. Mania may be a burst of esteem needed to save our life. A volcano can be destructive to human life, but its activity is necessary to create new land. After the lava cools, other people can walk on that land too that weren't there before the eruption. We are creating territory in consciousness by living through mania when we don't repress and ignore it. Eventually, others can walk in it too, without having to go through it themselves.

PERMISSION TO BREAK THE TABOO AND GLORIFY MANIA

"Mania is art plus defiance."

- Chris Cole

Sharing Mania, Actually

When I got a bipolar diagnosis in the psych ward in 2011, I knew I couldn't talk about my actual experiences. Anything I might say would only be further proof validating my visit to the inpatient unit. Since then, I've had many signs that I should speak up. I've been quiet about this for so long. I've now given myself permission to make meaning out of my experiences, and now I'm permitting myself to share it. In mania, we are privileged with the magic and the mysterious, along with the well-known costs. Mania can be an opportunity to explore these parts of the spectrum of human potential that everyone has, but few contact in ways prolific enough to dive deep. Parallels and overlaps between human potential and mania are easy to find but are awaiting philosophic and pragmatic application. The emphasis on the medical model and what's wrong overshadows the human potential in mania. It rarely asks if anything seemed right. The medical model is design for acute care and outpatient care but not to harvest the positives after the emergency part is over. After my diagnosis, it took me years to make peace with the mental health system. We don't need to argue, convince, explain, prove, or justify our experiences. Yet, here we'll start to look and speak of them in unlimited ways so our experiences and ideas can enter the market of human attention. I don't know about you, but I'm sitting on a ton of content. The system is designed to deal with us via our illness, and illness is always bad. If we identify predominantly with having an illness, we then think we are bad. This cannot be the right starting point or approach. It's up to us to play, have fun, experiment, test, wonder, and figure out the rest of our life for ourselves. I hope it becomes clear that we don't need permission. At the same time, it can help to explicitly give ourselves permission, if not now, by the end of this book.

It's up to us to extrapolate and apply the positives, potential, and possibilities. We don't have to wait and can start now if we are willing to do the work of putting are awareness and attention on playing with words, meaning, and perspectives. Let's be clear. We are human beings with potential and possibilities. Let's make our language, identifiers, and descriptors reflect this. We can distinguish ourselves beyond triggers, signs and symptoms, breakdown, and crisis. Mania is a type of breakthrough. It's time to see our experiences added into the descriptions, stories, and scriptures of transformation. Maybe after all our explorations, we conclude that we are just mentally ill and are no worse off.

Self-Recognition is Key for Releasing Potential

Psychology talks of self-esteem, self-acceptance, and self-compassion to resist negativity. What about self-recognition of our potential? When we are in our potential, there is little need to accept or have compassion for ourselves because we know who we are and what our potential is. We are creating faster than any chance of self-berating. People who self-recognize their true potential and possibilities get called grandiose by those who live at the level of self-esteem, self-compassion, and self-acceptance. And there's nothing wrong with that, but there's nothing wrong with being in a place where we need to self-recognize. The need to self-recognize hasn't yet been recognized. Mania maps our possibilities and gifts us the ability to recognize our potential because we live in the energy and territory. We see it and know it by doing it and living it. Self-recognition can only be lived, not conceptualized about. It's time to self-recognize this for ourselves.

Can we begin to map out a manic cosmology, as in how we see the world? Though mania is not the only way of mapping potential, if we've had mania, it's a good place to start. We can find clues about the meaning of our experiences by framing them with human potential lenses and perspectives. Right now, our primary lens is illness, so we start from a low vantage point that's hard to see beyond. We've been oppressed. Here, we're going to put the illness lens aside to try on lenses and perspectives of our own making. But we won't start from there. Maybe we feel some powerful identities or perspectives when we have mania. Maybe they feel real or at least possible. Can we try characteristics from those identities and apply them in daily life?

Maybe it feels far-fetched because we are disqualified from using certain phrases as soon as we are labeled bipolar. Saying things like, "I am eternal, infinite possibilities living in Heaven on Earth" or "We are all God living a human experience" are a sign of illness. Yet many religions and new age spiritualities insist the above claims to be true. Every spiritual seeker is attempting to live lives "as God" or "of God." Bipolar disorder means our insights are grandiose and that we have no insight into our illness. There was a time when people were burned at the stake and killed for heresy if they didn't bow down to religious, government, and now scientific authority. To boot, we're lighting the fire ourselves with self-stigma and losing sight of how our life is at stake. Doctors who spend a decade and thousands and thousands of dollars paying for their educational buy-in easily inoculate our consciousness with the illness paradigm. After all, they've paid to be experts.

In a manic state, what we say we're experiencing, we experience as real. We act as if our perceptions are genuine because we experience them that way. As bipolar people, we sometimes get to the point where we feel like Jesus, Buddha, the Dalai Lama, Mother Theresa, Shiva, or other Enlightened beings. If we 'come out' as some human conceptualized version of "God," it's because the feeling is innervating every fiber of our being. We aren't reading that we are as "God" in one of the many new age books or old religious texts and agreeing with it conceptually. We feel it beyond human conceptualization, but we don't know how to explain it to ourselves or others without using metaphors of these conceptualizations. Most traditional religions only allow for verbal agreement of being one with "God," even if the text implies otherwise. The funny thing is, no one can tell you if you've seen your true nature or not, though they can pull out all the stops to gaslight you into believing you're just crazy. We experienced we are a part of Gaia, a being and organism much bigger than ourselves.

In mania, it's an actual, living, pragmatic ecstasy. Maybe it's only temporary, but so is reading it in a book. I've said to myself the next coming out will be coming out as "One." Maybe it can only be a self-realized fact that we must self-recognize for ourselves. Instead of celebrating our temporary realization, we're captured and medicated. To the mainstream, it's an emergency to get the individual to forget their one-realization as soon as humanly possible, no matter how inhumane. A realized being no longer belongs to society, family, the economy, or any other system or structure. It becomes convenient to explain it away as illness. Then we are allowed to hope we can erase everything we experienced from our consciousness and go back to normal—as if that's the ideal.

In society, as long as any superhuman feelings remain conceptual, it's okay. Or a few gurus are allowed to be enlightened, especially if they remain isolated in a cave and don't buy a ranch. In both cases, the order of the consensus is maintained. It's not something to be experientially felt-sensed-embodied and actually lived out by a mere mortal. We aren't supposed to get a taste of immortality. It's a forbidden zone hidden within us and a part of our consciousness we aren't allowed to access because we'd be a powerful and cooperative humanity. There are no profits there, though there are many prophets.

If you expresses magic joy for no reason, the reason must be madness. In mania, the temporary celebration of realizing the ecstasy of the unique impossibility of being the human being we happen to be, could land us in the psych ward, branded with a lifelong mental illness label. We are invalidated. We can't express the joy of being human. It's not safe to show ourselves. We aren't allowed to love ourselves unconditionally. If we have a valid reason to act happy, like inebriation, buying a new car, or drug induction, then it's okay because the happiness will soon pass. It's not innate: it's rational and has a cause. What has a beginning has the end needed for endless seeking. Humanity is addicted to reasons and causes because the mathematics of what makes our psyche tick has been calculated to work against us. We get sideways looks for discovering the causeless celebration of the love of being a loving human beyond measure.

After mania, we find out our experiences are outside the allowable limits. We are not allowed to think, speak, or act in manic ways. We aren't allowed to explore and create who we are, moment by moment. We aren't allowed to be spontaneous, original, or different than how others remember our personality is supposed to be. We are tethered to the past and live in a prison of it. That's why it's taboo to speak positively about our mania experiences. It's safer to remain a mime of programs and a parrot of our past. It's okay to repeat what someone else said but not okay to come up with original ideas and thoughts on the fly. As a humanity, we've devolved our brains to only be able to handle very little new information without discomfort. And we wonder why we remain bored in a sea of new information, meaning, and beauty from nature and humanity.

It's considered shameful to go beyond our mediocre self and realize the ecstasy of being human. We're not supposed to remember the natural, innate joy snatched away from us in childhood. Finding our original source of joy within is a sin. And we feel like we've sinned after mania. We need to suspend our belief in our defectiveness and ponder the peak and peek of joy we discovered. We should ponder the source of life. We should realize our brain can miraculously metamorphose beyond the encrusted shell of the ego. The ego tells false stories about who we are, and we live in these low vibration stories. Programs are like viruses that mess up the software of who we truly are. Programs live in place of us, like parasites living off their host. We want others to know what we discovered so that they can discover it too to change their story.

Mania is Like Riding a Bike – You Never Forget

When we do talk about ourselves, we are taught to share our stories in the framework of our journey through mental illness. We enter the domain of stigma, a game we know too well. We teach others that we have a mental illness called bipolar disorder, and inadvertently commit an act of self-stigma. If we dare to share experiences that felt spiritual or positive, we have to say it was just our illness and we were just grandiose. We are afraid of the positive aspects because then we are glorifying an illness, which is contradictory. We make our experiences taboo and caught in a catch-22 of silence. When we talk about ourselves in the illness framework we are congratulated, called brave and courageous, and told we have "insight." We are hoping to avoid discrimination and prejudice. We take ownership and identify the cause within the biology of ourselves. Yet all the above factors are psychosocial. We are given chemical medications to suppress psycho-bio-social-spiritual energy. We've had a non-ordinary, ecstatic, or peak experience, and past trauma, and now we get an extra-large dose of oppression. And we pseudo-willingly take this on ourselves. Is it that the consensus world can't dare to entertain extraordinary potential because of the risk of loosening the collective belief in mediocrity and conformity? We live in a mediocracy, a society where extraordinary is suppressed into the exception and not the rule. If our extraordinary isn't oppressed, we don't need rulers. That's why to maintain the social order, we must self-stigmatize and believe others are stigmatizing us for our illness. We waste so much energy in this linguistic game.

Just as we never forget how to ride a bike, we never forget what it's like to be in mania. After being labeled with an illness and flung to the bottom of the social order, we're encouraged to self-deprecate and beg for tolerance. We take it on because we are captured and re-educated in a vulnerable crisis state. We ask others not to stigmatize the self-denigrated and oppressed version of ourselves we passively and painfully adopted. When we self-stigmatize, we reinforce the illness programming within ourselves and the collective. We parrot our story of illness and play victim to what we've been hypnotized into believing about ourselves. What happens if we withdrawal the buy-in in our consciousness after many years of oppression? It's important to withdrawal in this way and draw up a new consciousness before endeavoring to withdraw from other aspect of psychiatry. We need a new foundation.

In my experience, I've never self-stigmatized, nor thought that others should not stigmatize me, and I've experienced "stigma" three times in 10 years. Those few times, I realized they couldn't know me. I never absorbed or installed the stigma program—it's not a fun game. The whole stigma thing brings in self-justification and searching for acceptance. Instead I chose to love my brain by learning. Most of us play the stigma game because we easily forget how awesome we are or can be. The Oxford Dictionary defines stigma as "a mark of disgrace associated with a particular circumstance, quality or person" and we don't have to buy into this game. We need to unlearn it if we did, not by focusing on it, but by withdrawing our attentional resources and applying them to making our own game. We can look at what we saw when the veil was lifted instead of feeling ashamed of it.

We need to devote less words to parroting what we've been told about our lack of potential via diagnosis and share what we know about potential from our experience. Which way has a better chance of manifesting our potential? There are billions of people on this planet. We don't need to convince the whole world that it's okay to have a mental illness. We need to convince ourselves that we know something about human potential because we lived it. The illness in all of humanity is that we've been trained to miss out on our potential. And when we forget to remember our potential, we feel like something is missing. Looking for stigma and being angry about it is another way we are distracted into wasting our sacred attention on low energy and vibration matters. We are reinforcing the illness factor in our life. This can only attract more low vibration events that make us feel stigma. Let's create our own, more fun games.

Shifting your self-focus towards potential and possibilities breaks the taboo of speaking positively about mania. Addressing stigma is confirming a dying paradigm. We can make the paradigm dwindle in our life through our efforts to stop remembering it and then forget it. We can drop stigma from our consciousness when we no longer compare ourselves to those yet to metamorphose. Then we have more energy for what matters, and we can create our lives. What if there were a state of mind or mindset called "self-fulfilling" that went beyond self-acceptance, self-esteem, or self-compassion? Do we have to accept the defective self we take on with a diagnosis? Do we resist it and build self-esteem? Do we sit in self-compassion for ourselves because we are defective? These mindsets are based on lack and fear. In the mindset of self-fulfillment, with each new perception and moment, we are full, and that is all. Each moment fulfills us, and we move from one fulfillment to the next. We are in a state where the Universe can fulfill our order—the order of being human and our unique dreams. We want to exist, yet we forget how, until mania. In mania, we are what we've been looking for, so we live life from a state of fullness.

Be a Bipolar Bodhisattva?

Imagine breaking the taboo of embracing positives from mania and applying them to ourselves now? We need to give ourselves permission, and we need to do it now. I proclaim I'm a bipolar "Bodhisattva." According to Mahayana Buddhism, a Bodhisattva is a person who reaches enlightenment but instead of staying there in eternal bliss (and maybe leaving the body), returns to daily life to help others. What if the mental illness system is actually a Western world portal needed to return from the dimension of mania to the material paradigm? It's our landing pad back to the mainstream world. The portal back is a rough ride, and we can come back looking tired and disheveled, but it's the best we've got. Until now, the awareness of the system's function as a portal has been double-blind. The mental health system is unaware it's providing a portal back from touching enlightenment for potential Boddhisatva's. They can't and don't know where we went and what metamorphosis took place, and the reverse metamorphosis required to come back. We need the help of the system to get back. When we look at it this way and understand it ourselves, we don't need to be afraid. A bipolar diagnosis is just a clever disguise. It's not an easy rhythm of life and we need to create our own identity. If we don't, we could be mental patients forever, and the children behind us to. Just like the people institutionalized before us, we need to push the limits of our chemical and memetic institutionalization. The mental illness identity is rock bottom, so it's a starting point. Maybe mental illness is one way the Universe creates more Bodhisattvas?

Speaking in a positive light about experiences in mania is labeled "glorifying" or "romanticizing" the manic state. Yet speaking negatively about ourselves, symptoms, or suffering is encouraged as "ending stigma," as strength, courage, and hope. I'm not the first to argue for extra-ordinizing bipolar. Many have done amazing inspiring work comparing emotional crisis to spiritual emergency, extraordinary states, and many other perspectives. I recommend reading as much as you can, enhancing your map of perspectives. Sean Blackwell has an amazing series on YouTube called "Bipolar or Waking Up." I've watched it twice and I highly recommend it.

EntertainmentMania! and Consumerism

Many movies, like psychological thrillers, and songs use aspects and symptoms of mania, psychosis, craziness, and bipolar to generate entertainment and profit, whether it is a deliberate portrayal of someone with a mental health condition or not. There is a double standard where the entertainment industry can throw around the words, symptoms, and themes for entertainment purposes and profit, where the same in real life would be mental illness—and it's not pretty or entertaining. Yet we are grandiose when we describe the positive aspects we feel and perceive from our own real, embodied living experience. Again, unless it's carefully controlled and spoon-fed as 'fictional' entertainment to the masses, creating profits for the film industry, it's not okay. But I can't candidly express what I'm experiencing in mania without building a case against myself to be tranquilized. I should be allowed to profit from my own experiences—energetically, meaningfully, and spiritually. Maybe people could listen to us and write movie scripts. That would be a better role than filling psychiatry's scripts. People experience altered states and non-ordinary experiences all the time, but we aren't encouraged to find our own silver linings. While we keep silent, our silver linings end up on the silver screen.

What if there were a traveling show of improvisational 'manics?' If the public saw what we could make possible when we aren't oppressed, it would change perception and eliminate stigma. It'd be like watching a magic show, but with manic people and not magicians. We should at least be granted our own reality TV show. Imagine if mania were seen as entertainment rather than illness. Imagine we were given the choice not to be medicated but we had to live in co-housing with other manic people. We might self-organize like social insects rather than be dissected and socially isolated. Maybe we'd co-harvest our manias. As crazy as it sounds, that might be a step up from the historical and present torture many of us endure via being psychiatrized. Humanity might learn a lot more about flow and creativity from a whole house of un-tranquilized people in mania, especially if we were supported by Shaman, mystics, and other visionaries. Instead, we learn more and more about mental illnesses. It'd be more fun to be in a big, beautiful house with some of my peers to demonstrate there are gifts, than be in a gaslighting, cold medical ward. Why not build a huge, safe playground for manic people to be creative and express while living in the upside of mania, rather than lock people in rooms on its downturn? Society isn't safe for people in mania, and if we knew there was a safe, encouraging place to go when manic, we'd go on our own accord. If you build it, they will come. Instead, we have the opposite. We have the psych ward, which everyone resists.

Most often we end up in the confines of the hospital involuntarily. After all, who in their right mind would want to go to a psych ward? Maybe we'd go to a safe manic playground, a welcoming haven designed for manics. I dream of building a safe space called "Glad Park," rather than "Mad Park," that is based on the premise of the famous "Rat Park" study. In the study, rats either lived in a rat heaven or rat hell. Rats that lived in poor conditions, rat hell, press a lever over and over to take drugs rather than eating food until they starved to death. Rats that lived in ideal conditions, rat heaven, didn't press a lever to self-medicate with illicit drugs, even though it was always available.[a] Glad Park would be for people in a manic state to stay safe while frolicking, flowing, and growing to capture and harvest the huge potential creative output of energy while being around others who are going through the same thing. It's a safe place to harvest the fruits of crazy–to collaborate and co-create with others. Just one wave of mania could yield information and meaning sufficient to seed and inspire the work of a person for an entire lifetime. If such a place existed, people in mania would want to go there to make the most of the gift of manic energy. We'd mitigate the risk of wasting the energy wandering in a society that doesn't understand and the situations we get into as a result. A person in mania is in a vulnerable state, and the world is a comparatively hostile place. At Glad Park, there would be supportive peers not in a manic state who would affirm the human potential and possibilities that people in mania are experiencing, rather than gaslighting the experience with psychiatric memes, as happens in the psych ward. There would be creative tools to capture and harvest the download of information.

By the time we get to the psych ward, we may be in a bad state, but that's because we received no support for the positive aspects of our experience before it was too late. Society has no place for people lost and stuck in a positive, possible, potential state. It has many places for people who are depressed, angry, or have commit crimes. Psychiatry waits for us to crash and then we get committed. If we created a place where manics would gladly turn themselves in, part of the psych ward paradigm would wither away. Why isn't there a 'happy ward' if elation is part of the 'illness'? The space would be perfectly co-designed for manic consciousness to flower. It would be 100% lived-experience approved. Just as Google and other corporations design their workspace conscientiously and meticulously for creativity and productivity, so would Glad Park. Glad Park also frames mania in a positive way. It's for people in a mood or extreme state of being elated to be alive and live in those possibilities for that time. People in that space need a unique place to go. People in elated and ecstatic states need to be cared for, kept safe, and cultivated.

Where else besides the entertainment industry is it currently okay to use the word "mania" and related terms and themes in positive ways? In another example, the word "mania" is used religiously in marketing to spruce up product names, tag lines, and generate more sales. I recently saw a product called "Ultra Violet Manic Panic" for bright purple hair color, "crazy salmon roll" for sushi, and a store called "Dollar Mania." Now that you've read this, my guess is you'll find hundreds of examples in your everyday life. I don't think they use the word "mania" because they want us to look away or run in the other direction. They use it because of the association of ecstatic excitement, mystery, and craziness—and it sells. They put manic traits, traits which belong to all of humanity, in advertising and marketing. They've been taken from us.

This is most apparent if mania actually happens to you. Then you'll be marketed and sold to the pharmaceutical industry and psychiatric assembly line. It's acceptable to use manic traits if you are a business with something to sell to consumers. What about mania as a state of buying back in to being who we really are or could be? When a human is in the state of mania, we are being marketed and sold our original ecstatic beingness back to ourselves from the Universe. It's a marketing algorithm of the Universe of our original trajectory. Missing this is a tragedy.

Maybe when someone becomes manic in public, the following scenario should unfold: Everyone's hair turns bright purple. They gather around the manic person for entertainment by the event of freely flowing, spontaneous, creative originality in ecstasy, and eat crazy sushi off plates from Dollar Mania. But human mania isn't marketed that way. Instead, we are led to the psych ward. More and more people are being trained with the psychiatric lens.[b] Meanwhile, entertainment and marketing can use the word mania and its implications to make movies for us to watch and sell stuff for us to buy. Yet it's taboo for me, a person with living experience of mania, to sell the state of mania and the products of it as something positive, not even to myself. And I'm not against anyone using crazy, mania, or bipolar as descriptive words for conversational, commercial, or entertainment purposes. I would like my state of mania to be included in the positive conversation. Crazy means awesome, fun, unbelievable, wow, etc. And that's what mania is! That's why I started saying positive things to myself about mania. No matter what happened after mania, that doesn't change that I experienced much of it as awesome. I discovered that I'm awesome, even if I don't always feel it. We all are, but our attention has been diverted.

Speaking of diverted attention, ever notice how people in commercials often act over the top, like they're a bit manic? We need to reclaim the excitement and life altering power of mania as a positive process, not to be feared or shunned. It has exciting connotations everywhere in our fabricated, consensus world, except I'm not supposed to identify with it that way. Let's declare immediately from this point forward, BipolarMania also has exciting connotations when someone goes manic and lives as themselves beyond fabrications. We need to watch their show as they step onto their body-stage. We need to re-realize our human potential. What takes the place of marketing? The only thing we're missing out on is here and now. There's nothing we need to do. Change from where you look at things and look at this moment now. Otherwise, we are looking at an illusion from an illusion. If we could see, everything would change in an instant, like we woke up from a nightmare.

Everyone Wants It, No One Gets it, Some are Touched

Dare I say, in its purest form, everyone wants mania. Anyone who alters their consciousness with substances, food, or entertainment wants to escape the limited monkey mind. We all want to live in the unlimited magic mind. With all the profits derived from making products or services to get into altered states, the possibility of free access to extraordinary states is provocative. Manics have non-volitional, free access to the altered state of mania, and it's not going away. Once mania makes contact, we know our unlimited nature, and we can't forget. We may not be able to control when mania calls, but we can be prepared for when it happens. When we feel limited and experience inner conflict between what is and what should be, we don't know it, but we want mania. We want energy to go beyond the conflict into a state of creation. That's the only way to live beyond conflict. Normal is a low energy state.

In a paper called *Positive Traits in the Bipolar Spectrum: The Space between Madness and Genius* by Tiffany A. Greenwood, has the right idea:

> Studies evaluating positive aspects and character strengths associated with bipolar disorder are aligned with the growing interest in research on the impact of positive psychological traits on health… Positive traits of spirituality, empathy, creativity, realism, and resilience are frequently observed in bipolar individuals… By gaining a better appreciation for the positive aspects of mental illness and exploring methods to enhance these traits, we may improve clinical outcomes… Current practice in psychiatry is geared more towards controlling the symptoms of bipolar disorder, rather than understanding a patient's true needs and potential capabilities.[19]

This scientific research is on the right track towards addressing our true needs and capacities. Bipolar has a steady worldwide prevalence rate.[20] Could it be a process of nature? A necessity? I'm speaking candidly and unapologetically to make prophets out of us, because we are creating profits for others by remaining silent. By calling it mental illness we block ourselves from trying to understand for ourselves because we must rely on the mental illness tradition and its preachers. The thought of mental illness locks away the mysteries. Bipolar is a gag order. I'm not the psychiatrically constructed version of myself. The psychiatrically constructed version is a disguise, and it covers over my original blueprint. In our game, we are building a visionary mystery, not a psychiatric history. I speak openly about bipolar with AWE-FULL-EYES—eyes full of awe. Bipolar gave me new eyes. These eyes renew themselves. This ability, as well as other bipolar traits, have permeated all aspects of my life.

I watched a program called "A Bipolar Expedition" and two quotes stuck out to me. The first: "In your mania there is no rhyme or reason to anything. You just live in your fantasy world until you come down with a bump."[21] The second: "People pay thousands for drugs to get where you are and never quite get there. It's something that's better than taking any drugs. You are completely flying differently naturally."

Ron Unger is a clinical social worker and therapist in the field who brings understanding to the possible benefits of altered states and psychosis. In general, talk therapy isn't provided to people with psychotic disorders as there is a belief in the nonsensicality and dangerousness of entertaining psychosis and its ideas. Unger cleverly refers to the assumption that engaging psychotic content is too risky as "Risky risk avoidance." He brings up several important points worth noting in his course *CBT for Psychosis*:

- *Contesting what things mean and creating some chaos can be part of overthrowing an existing unhelpful rigidly held system of meaning or rigidly held anything.*

- *Illness = no way to make sense of it or integrate it, thus it must be repressed or eliminated. But that means missing the metaphorical message and if the message is important to the person's psyche, it will keep finding ways to express itself despite any attempts at repression.*

- *We also sometimes need to recover from the limitations from our version of sanity.*

- *The process can be beneficial and can come back with something that is beneficial to the wider society.*

- *If it's put into clear expression, then it may no longer need to express it in a psychotic way.[22]*

I've never heard anything like that from the psychiatric system. Unger's points lend further weight to the action of giving ourselves permission to break the taboo of speaking in positive terms about our experiences. He is a great thought leader and resource through his website recoveryfromschizophrenia.org

THE IMPORTANCE OF THE RE-UNCOVERY PROCESS

"What if the worst thing that happened to you becomes the best thing that happened to you?"

- Dr. Joe Dispenza

When Creativity is Salient, Salience is Creative

We need more creativity in our world. Medications can repress creative traits. Should the goal be to continuously medicate the creative state into submission? Can we give ourselves permission to re-claim our creative mission? Collectively, we can create a wisdom tradition and philosophy of Re-Uncovery. That doesn't mean we don't participate in recovery. On the contrary. Remember, recovery and Re-Uncovery go together. While recovery helps deal with distressing symptoms so we can be practical, Re-Uncovery harvests and navigates eustressing signs of magic, so we can achieve what we thought impossible. Manic events starting in 2011 until present have never left me and continue to hold a great significance in my being. I can't forget the mystery. I can't forget the magic. Because of mania, I know reality can work in mysterious ways and I am of the mystery. When we know who we are and come alive, illness marketing dies. Then the scientific method can no longer capture the methods behind madness.

We need more accounts from all parts of the spectrum in addition to the overemphasis on hedonism, violence, and sexcapades. The picture of mania is skewed. This thought is supported by extrapolating to the emerging understanding of dopamine's role in both the value coding system and salience system.[k] Put simply, dopamine's function in the salience network is related to seeing, finding, and creating meaning. Dopamine in the value system is related to pleasure. Humanity is yet to reach the critical mass needed to have the fulfillment associated with seeing meaning for its own sake. In commerce, fulfillment is completing the order. In consciousness, fulfillment is co-creating the perception with our essence. When we subjectively complete a perception, we fulfill a different order of the world. We get tripped up by the exploratory salience network because we are programmed to the value system, which is the kind of consciousness we are advertised from birth.

We need to glorify the rich spectrum of mania as a peak experience. Not everyone experiences hyper-hedonism as a part of mania. Not everyone acts violent. Not everyone experiences downloads of information and meanings coming from an unfamiliar source. Yet this is an untold part we have yet to fully unfold. The well-known characteristics are the well-known through media, entertainment, psychiatry, and our own self-reports. The traits that get us in trouble are overrepresented in the literature. Just because a flight has turbulence doesn't mean the whole trip wasn't worth it. If we go on a trip, we don't just talk about the turbulence when we get back. Yet that's what we've been convinced to do when we touch down. The positive stuff that could help to outweigh the negative and justify some of the extreme costs is missing. We need more literature on the subtle, salient aspects too. When we understand the significance of mania as an open portal and bring intentionality to it, we can reduce the harm of hedonism of an inflated value coding system and move towards transcendent understanding through the salience system. I'm more interested in manic-idea-sex. Mania can either provide the energy to open us up to a new dimension, or the energy to augment our ego structures. Inevitably, both mechanisms lead to the destruction of the ego, by either disengagement or inflation. Both hedonism and grandiosity create drama that helps ensure we eventually return to consensus level consciousness because they inflate to obvious proportions. The aspects of mania or psychosis that led us to the psych ward are the ones we need to grow out of in favor of all the rest. There are many aspects of mania psychiatry doesn't know about and never will. There are many you can only know by living it. And that's the part we are excavating, instead of the usual evading.

Mutually Exclusively Guiding Curiosity or
Fear of the Elusive

When we get curious about mania, we can take a page from its book, and learn to be and feel awesome more often. When we fear mania, look away, close our eyes, and cross our fingers that it'll never happen again, we fail to learn and fail to adapt. Mania is our natural-excited-about-life state that we are born with. It's stripped away as we grow up. If it were never taken away, we'd have adapted to the higher-level energy state, and our bodies would be more capable of handling it. Throughout life, our bodies would have built the physiology and anatomy to go along with the energy. There would be no mania. Mania is an energetic bridge of the gap to what would have been, and what could still be, as we see in mania. We must gather the pointers from mania to discover the keys, because what we've gone through is important and valuable to us and culture.

Some of us already know the value of the manic state and we can be valuable guides. We can blaze the trails of the ecstatic subjectivity and build a scaffolding of uncharted context. The trouble is outside observers of mania need to have a bit of faith. Why faith? They need to ask us different questions than they've ever asked. For starters, re-frame the psych ward intake form and ask us about our journey. Don't just ask if we had special messages from the TV and check a box. Ask us what the messages were and write them down for us so we can read them later. Ask us what it's like to journey to inner heights like astronauts back from a space mission. We will have lots to share. Don't just ask us about the path we took to crash back to Earth. Approach us with a wondering gaze and we can pass on a wondrous mystery. I'd like non-experiencers to ask awesome, positive, mystical questions and have a dialogue with us so we can share and unfold our meaning. Soon, when we say we had a non-volitional mania, others will be in awe and want to talk with us. We will shift from appearing weary to being wise. Gather the evidence you need to justify showing us extraordinary care and compassion. Ask us for our insights from our journey. Don't try to convince us to have insight into our illness. First, the hidden illness is the lack of communication that has given rise to the chasm between the natural world and the artificial world. We can fill the gap together by having dialogue, because mania is a gift that sees and goes beyond the veil. Don't sacrifice us for the comfort of the status quo because we are very uncomfortable with it. We can share the truth of what we experienced. Hear, don't just listen when we are trying to point out something that would be otherwise unnoticeable.

Psychiatry Has Done Us a Big Favor

The diagnosis "bipolar" is a key word we can use to easily find each other and create a self-selected neuro-tribe based on living experience. We can call it whatever we want after that. They've brought us together so we can figure it out together, and we can move on. Where psychiatrists see symptoms of an illness, I see signs of a neuro-tribe with the key to a source code. We can build the scaffolding and move on together. Now we can speak and communicate in new ways with each other. We already have years of experiences: we just needed permission. We can crowd out the old paradigm by adding in the new meaning within us that is missing, suppressed. The illness model will be a small fraction of how we make meaning out of our experiences. The illness paradigm is a holding pattern, just like a plane waiting until it's safe to land. We've been waiting for the time to create a new paradigm. Reality is emerging to be in alignment with our potential and possibilities. In the future, others won't have to fall from mania into the psych system because the whole world will be a higher vibration when we contribute our missing meaning.

What Dr. Daniel Siegel called the "consilient" findings of science, are those often independently discovered truths that have common ground.[23] Bipolar also has consilient findings with science. We can discover truths with our perception that science has also confirmed with experiments. We can see how some of the weird discoveries of science relate to mania. What we uncover in mania isn't because of science; they are independently discovered. We can look at this the other way around too. The discoveries in experiments in the realm of human potential can be applied to some aspects of mania. The findings are consilient because there is common ground and because there is common ground, we can use them to build our understanding of ourselves outside the medical model.

We need other information from more sciences besides psychiatry to help explain and understand mania. When we understand how weird reality is, we see that our perceptions in mania are not that far off. Weird things happen all around us in daily life; we just don't usually notice. When we act weird in mania we are in contact with the weirdness of reality. Maybe it's strange not to notice how weird reality is. Scientists say most of the Universe is non-detectible in the form of dark energy and matter because their mathematics says it must exist.[24] Science can't detect it with their instruments. Stephen Hawking said before he died that the Universe is holographic and projected from a deeper reality.[25] Quantum physicists used to think quantum effects only happened at very tiny scales. Now they have studies that show quantum effects happen on the macroscopic scale in flocks of birds.[26] Experiments in quantum physics are looking for quantum effects at the macro scale of everyday life. But what if the brain could speed up, access more energy, and energize new circuits to see quantum effects with our own eyes? I think that's part of what happens to us in mania—sometimes, our brain goes quantum, and we can access quantum events in daily life. The old paradigm is Newtonian. The new paradigm is quantum, and it's about possibilities and perhaps impossibilities.

Shall We Too Revere Mania?

This process shall be revered rather than repressed. After all, we are thrust into a hyperdrive state of consciousness with no choice. Mania puts our brains and bodies at risk to gather these clues, insights, and new meaning. We are non-volitional psychonauts, and our journeys shall not be for naught. It's a waste of the energy of the Universe. We lose most of our insights and never end up contributing to culture. Many of us see the same themes or things, and if we all speak up together, to each other, we can create some amazing ripples and resonance. Are our weird 'symptoms' actually signs of a weird world, an emerging new paradigm, other dimensions of reality, parallel worlds, or quantum mechanics taking hold in our brain, mind, and consciousness? Or just an illness?

Illness is how we are treated, not who we are or what we've experienced. We aren't treated with compassionate empathy when we are in a crisis. We are supposed to be messengers, mystics, Shamans, seers, and psychics. There are so many more roles to step into and paths that are possible. The world isn't meant to have 2-6% of the world with mental illnesses called "bipolar disorder" and "schizophrenia." The world is meant to have 2-6% of people who are "visionaries," "intuitives," or "seers." If this were so, many of the world's problems would be solved from seeing from a higher vantage point. If more of us were embodying our true potential and taking a new role here on Earth, it would be a much more livable world for all of us. There'd be little depression compared to the amount plaguing the population, consuming entire lives and killing others. If 2% can own 98% of the wealth on the planet, I propose that the 2% that are seers can reveal the true wealth of the planet and tip the scales to take back our lives and live our dreams and possibilities. We can reveal the oneness and harmony that's been overwritten. But there is fear of the trans-conscious state and of people who suspend their personality to glean alternate information. We need faith. We need trust that maybe we see something that most people can't. We need care and compassion to sort it out. Our dreams and possibilities are happening now; we just don't have the energy or the eyes to see. Few really listen to us. Instead, we are locked away, medicated, and re-educated.

Chapter 2

PATHOLOGICAL IDEAS TO CROWD OUT

CARRY ON LIKE A THRIVER – BUT FIRST A CRITIQUE

"Like racism and sexism, mentalism infects its victims with the belief in their own inferiority, which must be consciously rooted out."

- Judi Chamberlain

Do We Have Time to Wait?

Bipolar is associated with creativity, artistry, spirituality, leadership, and more. There are no therapies designed to support us to augment and utilize our gained strengths and abilities. These are our self-proclaimed positive-positive symptoms. Advocates and educators like Ron Unger, David

Lukoff, Emma Bragdon, Katie Mottram, and Sean Blackwell have walked between paradigms and made it their life's work to bring light.

Many people find benefits in the medical model, including myself. I've had 99% positive experiences in the psych system, even though the system is limited in what it has to offer. I take medications as a compromise to keep my feet on the ground. I am grateful that the mental health system has been instrumental in my journey, especially the clubhouse model. I've had a few bad experiences, but in retrospect, it could be that elements of the dark night of the soul were playing out in the psych ward, perhaps not necessarily because of it.

The system is slowly changing in the right direction, but we don't have time to wait. The traditional approach could do better by being more lived-experience informed. Hopefully, it will include "self-directed services" soon, where we get a budget and choose services in a free market based on our own unique goals rather than in a preselected set of services that we either fit into or we don't. Until then, it's impossible not to mention some of the system's downfalls in the context of this book. Being part of the system, I lived through the limitations in the context and meaning I was given to frame my experiences. It was up to me to expand my understanding. I can re-contextualize that by saying the way the system lacks imagination has inspired my exploration of the territory beyond it and influenced the creation of this book. I've even come to see the mental health system as designed to hold us and deprive us of meaning, since we are meant to create the meaning ourselves. If the system gave us rich meaning, they would deprive us of figuring it out on our own. It may be possible that psychiatrists use harsh terms like "bipolar with psychotic features" to leave the rest up to us.

A Thought Experiment – What if the Psych System? Vs. the Psych System Does What Now?

Imagine if there were a perfect system that handed all the manic insights to us on a gold platter. Would we learn anything for ourselves? I propose diagnosis as an invitation to participate in transforming "insanity" back to a transformation process. It's only insanity when we keep repeating that it's all just insanity, thus doing the same thing over and over and expecting different results. At the same time, we can forgive them as they know not what they do, and tread past anger. We can see higher, farther, and deeper than they can at this moment, so maybe it's up to us to forgive first. The stigma can be dealt with through the 'sticks and stones' principle. Sticks and stones may break my bones, but I won't let being called mentally ill hurt me.

Most of the positive aspects of mania are beyond the scope and domain of the medical system especially regarding the human potential side of the spectrum. We need the energy of more people with lived experience exploring human potential—more than we use to fight stigma or advocate for system change. Although advocacy may be within our circle of influence, it may take decades to fundamentally change the system. We need a fundamental change now. We can explore our transformative potential for ourselves, and that's a fundamental change. The "clinical gaze"[27] may never catch up with what we can discover for ourselves with our own eyes. You've felt that oppression or diminishment when some doctors or clinicians look at you, right?

Another phenomenon to consider is gaslighting, which still occurs in subtle and not-so-subtle ways. According to Wikipedia, gaslighting is a form of psychological manipulation in which a person or a group covertly sows seeds of doubt in a targeted individual or group, making them question their memory, perception, or judgment.[28] There is even a section for gaslighting in the psychiatric context on the Wikipedia page:

> Gaslighting has been observed between patients and staff in inpatient psychiatric facilities. In a 1996 book, Dorpat claimed that "gaslighting and other methods of interpersonal control are widely used by mental health professionals as well as other people" because they are effective methods for shaping the behavior of other individuals. He noted that covert methods of interpersonal control such as gaslighting are used by clinicians with authoritarian attitudes, and he recommended instead more non-directive and egalitarian attitudes and methods on the part of clinicians, "treating patients as active collaborators and equal partners."[28]

We can take one step further and consider menticide, which is "the systematic effort to undermine and destroy a person's values and beliefs, as by the use of prolonged interrogation, drugs, torture, etc., and to induce radically different ideas."[29] We go to the psych ward with certain ideas and leave with drugs and a diagnosis. A friend in Russia told me a psych ward she was in sometimes closed the bathroom facilities. A patient got desperate and did their business in front of it. This torture is part of the menticide that punishes different ways of thinking about and experiencing the world. The system employs its tactics until we are forced to put faith in their interpretations. We must build robustness in our maps, meanings, values, and beliefs, otherwise we'll undergo a form of mania menticide again and again.

Priming New Roles Beyond Changing the Narrative

When we accept only the narrative we get, we are dumbed down to the level of that narrative. Some of us will always defend ourselves as diseased, defective, or disabled. We should have informed consent before taking on the paradigm and all the beliefs that go with it. The idea that it's a lifelong illness will one day be weeded out in favor of a temporary transformative healing crisis when it's supported as such. As more of us become nodes of new understanding, we will have a ripple effect through our circle of influence, the morphogenetic field, and quantum hologram. We will create ripples to bridge to better possible futures in the next now. We report similar phenomena across our experiences and that can be taken as signs of oneness and signals of a transformative crisis that is to be expected as part of normal human experience. Maybe more people will feel permission to let go and transform instead of always trying to hold it together, sometimes until it's too late.

What else does it mean? In addition to advocacy for system change and peer work in the system that's thankfully already going on, we can share our collective learning with ourselves and each other. When we work towards integration and want to do something with our experience and exploration, we may find we need to create new roles that we can fill. Are you a medium? Are you psychic? You define yourself. You create your own identities. Everyone will do this in the future when identity is decentralized from organizations. We can also challenge the belief that we will get worse over time. Why settle for the system's goal of a "satisfactory quality of life" when we can live our extraordinary life beyond the limits of oppression? What would humanity say today if a group of people were put in insulin comas, dunked in ice baths, and had their brains mangled by an icepick through the eye? Society will see what's considered best practice today as barbaric in a short time. Many psych system experiencers now consider ECT and chemical lobotomies barbaric, though the clinicians see it as best practice. These so-called treatments are oppression and torture of those who don't fit societies mold to maintain social order and the status quo. Many people die because of these medical treatments, but we don't see the side effects acted out on TV commercials.

Stan Grof says in the book The Holotropic Mind:

> "Important lessons I've learned from the study of non-ordinary states of consciousness is the recognition that many conditions mainstream psychiatry considers bizarre and pathological are actually natural mechanisms of the deep dynamics of the human psyche. In many instances, the emergence of these elements into consciousness may be the organism's effort to free itself from the bonds of various traumatic imprints and limitations, heal itself, and reach a more harmonious way of functioning."[30]

Even with a place such as Glad Park, some people would still choose the psych ward. There is something calming about being in an abysmal place when I'm feeling terror, panic, and despair. It's congruent with my inner state to be in a small bed with a single sheet in a cold room. I feel terrible and the psych ward is just another reason to feel that way. When I start to feel better, I graduate to better circumstances. I get the right food at mealtime, to wear my own clothes, go outside, go for a hobble down the block, then go on an outing for two hours. Once discharged, it feels rewarding just to pay a bill online, drive my car, or get groceries. It's a colossal accomplishment to be free to put the pieces back together and get it together. I appreciate that I'm free to do the simple things as long as I don't think too deep.

Medications and the thought that it's "all just a mental illness" are enough to turn down the volume on uncertainty, stress, and chaos. A label does its job of boxing us in and lowering our potential energy to the mundane and routine. Our bandwidth of experience narrows so we don't get out of line and scare others. The mental health system doesn't address the illusory nature of mainstream reality. We see too much of what's possible. After mania, we have insight into our potential and possibilities. No one can take it away. Not even medication. We don't stop taking medication because we have an illness, we stop because we have possibilities. We saw them, lived them, and want to go back there. A lifelong awareness of our possibilities is engrained in our minds.

Imagine we aren't victims. It took me a couple of years to get over my anger at the psych system. I had a bad hospitalization where I was paternalistically given medications that I knew I wouldn't respond positively to. They wouldn't let me change to the psychiatrist on the ward who helped me twice before. Rather than receiving help, I was in a fight for my life. After that time, I was afraid of going back to the psych ward, and I built the strength and made plans to stay away from the hospital three times. Years later, I knew I'd gone too far into psychosis, and I needed the hospital as a way back. It was a portal. And I got a new start from square zero. Since it's meaningless overall, I could create meaning for myself with a blank slate. The system is not the audience for listening to our meanings. They have not the time nor the relevant lived experience.

ON PSYCHIATRIC SYSTEM CHANGE

"The ego wants closure, it wants a complete explanation. The beginning of wisdom, I believe is the ability to accept an inherent messiness in your explanation of what's going on because nowhere is it writ that human minds should be able to give a full accounting of creation in all dimensions in all levels."

- Terence McKenna

Let's Move

Many movements are working tirelessly to change the mental health system and seed necessary improvements. MindFreedom, The Icarus Project now the Fireweed Collective, the Open Dialogue Approach, the Brazilian Spiritus Hospitals, Emerging Proud/ Kind, Drop the Disorder, Mad Pride, Un-Recovery, and Spiritual Emergency/Emergence, to name a few. They have overlapping and unique themes, values, and actions. These movements share commonalities; they propose alternative frameworks and interpretations to the disease model. Our Re-Uncovery model framework also has different meanings and interpretations. We start with not knowing nor making assumptions. We explore and include elements of many approaches. It's up to us. The new paradigm and new parallel world are an undivided and non-violent step in consciousness. This step in consciousness "is the first step and the last step," as J. Krishnamurti often said when talking about freedom.[31] Freedom isn't in the future: it's now or never. And freedom in consciousness is required to live in the stream of life. When we shift into mania, we experience a radical change and feel exponentially more degrees of freedom in movement, behavior, and interaction. All because of a change in consciousness.

The psychiatric-biomedical system is paternalistic. We subordinate ourselves to the authority of psychiatry. Some alternative approaches question whether paternalism is necessary and could be harmful. Stigma comes from accepting the paternalistic narrative. What is little known is that self-stigma is an inner form of self-paternalism. We've taken on the paternalism of psychiatry, internalized it, and used it against ourselves. Can we take a step away from fighting the paternalism of the system and take a step in our consciousness to free ourselves of paternalism? We need to re-create our own inner space beyond the oppression and stigma we've faced. Oppression thrives on taking on and accumulating oppressive ideas and thoughts. These ideas and thoughts clog our brains and slow them down. Clogging up and slowing down the brain completes the loop, ensuring the continuing oppressive and paternalistic nature of the mind. This is a vicious cycle that wastes the energy we need to see clearly. In our natural state, our mind is not paternalistic, and it's free from oppressive mechanisms. How can life impress us now when we are oppressed by the past? We can shift our inner system to be a little bit manic all the time—in daily life. The solution isn't less mania, as we will come to see, it's more mania—more manic energy and manic traits.

On Disrupting Psychiatry

So how does attempting to change the mental health system take our attentional resources away from raising our consciousness? Do we need some balance? For this I will draw on work by Ron Unger[32] as well as a book called *Psychiatry Disrupted, Theorizing Resistance and Crafting the (R)Evolution*[4]. *Psychiatry Disrupted* helped me tease out distinctions I was unaware of and see where the approach in this book fits in. I've always wondered if I am "anti-psychiatry" or not. As it turns out, I'm not. In the book, the term "anti-psychiatry" means that first, there is no point to try to fix the mental health system, and second, any attempt to make the system better or fix it is an action that anti-psychiatry would not endorse[4]. Though I may see that using an inside-out process is much more fulfilling, I do participate in changing the system if the opportunity presents itself. A few years ago, I was on several committees in the health authority for mental health community redesign as a person with lived experience. Recently, I participated in a phone interview to give input on changing the procedure for informing psychiatric patients of their rights when involuntarily committed under the Mental Health Act. Participating in system change can't be more paradoxical than bettering the process of being involuntarily detained. Not only that, but I also take psychiatric medications: therefore, by default I'm participating in psychiatry every day when I swallow those pills. I agree with the brilliant wholistic psychiatrist Dr. Kelly

Brogan that when we are put on psychiatric medications, we aren't given true, informed consent on the risks and benefits[33]. In her book Freedom From Psychiatric Drugs, Chaya Grossberg says "Informed consent is knowing at least 20 other possible explanations for your experiences than the Western medical model so you are choosing which one to go with rather than accepting the one that pharmaceutical companies paid billions of dollars to put in front of your face in every corner of your world. For true informed consent, study models from all different cultures and times in history before consenting."

Medications are very difficult to taper off of. Iatrogenic effects, or withdrawal symptoms caused by habituation to the medications that present while attempting to taper off, are used as evidence for the often repeated, "see you need to stay on medications." Symptoms of withdrawal from the medications are taken as symptoms of illness. We aren't told that we likely won't ever be able to get off of the medications since our bodies become addicted to them and there is no support system to help us do so. I suppose the benefits are considered to outweigh the risks by psychiatrists, but there is no way to assess this on an individual biochemical basis. It's trial and error, and sometimes the error is death. Besides, they don't have to get informed consent when we can't refuse the medications in the case of involuntary committal anyway. By the time we've been informed of our rights, we're already drugged up, which makes it near impossible to enact our right to a second opinion or whatever other 'rights' we may have. Maybe psychiatrists need to take antipsychotics during their training, like law enforcement trainees have to experience pepper spray.

Ron Unger says Indigenous cultures go into altered states. It's encouraged because the risk to the individual is less than the potential benefit to the community. Additionally, the community elders and Shaman rally to fully support them.[34] We've never tried to find out if states of mania can benefit the community. Imagine if the community rallied to fully support individuals in mania to harvest the golden nuggets of information and insights. Our game is to harvest the lost benefits. We need to build our own system to not lose our gifts. We need to "treat" each other to the discoveries of each of us and create a culture of sharing. As we do, our perceived need for "treatment" will fade away. Not only that, but we can also support others so they can be the authors of their own lives. Ron Unger also poignantly says that "sanity is limited in what it has to offer" and that we must "nurture those who look outside sanity."[35]

Much of the sanity or madness is in our own words and use of language. Language is very powerful. I re-frame and re-language words to be in alignment with what I'm pointing at and what's possible. For example, I use the word "mad" less because of its association with anger, aggression, and violence. I think it's an old, outdated term that's had its day in my consciousness. I vibe with being glad about my ability to learn, create, and integrate meaning. I certainly agree with Ron Unger when he says:

> But many of those who have lived through the experience of being mad or psychotic did find something of value in their experience, something to be proud of. And the discovery of something positive in the experience is often understood to play an important role in the process of recovery from the disabling aspects of psychosis.[35]

Bipolar and psychosis *are* disabling, but am I inherently disabled? I prefer saying I have a 'perceived disability.' My diagnosis or label is informative for psychiatrists or people I share my recovery story with. I don't really know if I'm disabled or if I've lost certain abilities society labels as valuable in exchange for new ones. As much as there might be a disability perceived by the status quo, I am 'abilitated' in the manic world. I feel disabled according to, by, and from the social construction that we call the world. Sometimes I can feel the heavy, destructive energy that weighs us all down. I function better in lighter worlds. Medications are like gravity boots that keep my feet on the Earth. I've learned to walk in both worlds, and I can be a bridge to the other worlds.

On page 120 of *Psychiatry Disrupted*, an essay by A.J. Whithers says the following about disability and stigma:

> Like it or not, the disabled identity is not one that is within the control of most disabled people, and the experience of disabilities certainly is not. This is partly because disability (including impairment) is a social construction, and there are no fixed borders to determine who is and who is not disabled. You are disabled if you are constructed as disabled, and the stigma and subordination comes along with that.[36]

Although I said I have a perceived disability, I can't escape the fact that I'm being constructed as disabled, as if there are truly fixed boundaries, and what society calls important are valuable abilities. Here we are working and playing to change those perceived boundaries within ourselves and help us remember that we've already expanded beyond them.

Is this a human problem? A.J. Withers, in his essay *When Resisting Psychiatry is Oppressive* on page 122 of *Psychiatry Disrupted*, writes about the gay rights movement. Through the efforts of gay people, homosexuality was removed from the DSM, and gay people were no longer labeled as having a psychiatric illness, but as a minority group.[36] They managed to "un-psychiatrize" homosexuality. The DSM-5 continued to include a category for individuals who self-identified and sought help because they were distressed by being homosexual. Families could no longer commit members to psychiatric hospitals for being gay. It would be great if the DSM-5 only applied to bipolar as an illness if we self-identified it as disturbing to us. Then there'd be no 'lack of insight into our illness.'

This got me thinking, might bipolar people one day be a minority group in the community with unique needs and services, but not part of the psychiatric paradigm? Surprisingly, Whithers goes on to argue that people who are psychiatrized should not try to become un-psychiatrized because that is detrimental to the rest of the whole spectrum of the disability community. Of note, Whithers identifies as both physically and psychiatrically disabled. Even though I am psychiatrically labeled and disabled as well as being a non-heterosexual, I don't share the same view. Personally, I'm glad gay people fought for their freedom, and because of the efforts of those before me, I don't have two 'disabilities' in the DSM-5. Now transgender people are being liberated. I wouldn't want them to hold themselves back from their liberation because it lowers my chance of bipolar liberation. Not only that, but I also agree with J. Krishnamurti when he says if we change radically, it affects the whole consciousness of mankind.[37] So why wait? It's not so much a matter of changing the system as it's a problem of missing context. Adding the missing context will create the memetic pressure for the system to change.

Who is on the Right Track Regarding Disability Rights?

Not long after finishing my exploration of *Psychiatry Disrupted*, I received an email from madinamerica.com that included an article published by Robert Whitaker, the author of *Anatomy of an Epidemic*. Even while British Columbia is fast creating processes to make the involuntary hospitalization process "better" and more informative for the inpatient, Robert Whitaker writes of new information fresh from the World Health Organization regarding disability rights for all. He stated that in 2008, the UN Convention on the Rights of Persons with Disabilities (CRPD) states that the same rights and fundamental freedoms should be enjoyed by people with disabilities like everyone else.[c] It has been ratified by 181 countries, not including the USA. Whitaker says although the WHO doesn't specifically point out criticisms in the biomedical model, it connotes its failure. He says, "This WHO document, by urging societies to create services free of coercion and to enact laws and policies that prohibit such coercion, is supporting a radical change in global mental health services."[c] Regarding coercion, he quoted the WHO documents declarations of "...ensuring that human rights underpin all actions in the field of mental health, ... respecting their will and preferences in treatment, implementing alternatives to coercion."[c] Whitaker also illustrates how all this forced treatment gets justified: "In the biomedical model, people with severe 'mental illness' are said to suffer from anosognosia, a lack of insight into their illness, and this becomes the stated justification for forced hospitalization and treatment. This is what gives society and providers guardianship power over those with mental health issues and disabilities."[c] This is the ultimate catch-22.

So how do we get out of a catch-22? Can we wait for options like the Open Dialogue Approach where a team of 16 different clinicians is there to treat you and "attempt to promote the client's potential for self-exploration, self-explanation, and self-determination."[38] According to Robert Whitaker, there is a rising non-pharmaceutical paradigm for psychosis. Only 10-15% of people diagnosed with schizophrenia recover after 15 years on meds and people seem to deteriorate after four years on medication. The poor long-term outcomes mean the medicalized paradigm has largely failed.

Psychiatry Abolished?

Bonnie Burstow talks about the attrition model for withering away the mental illness model until it's abolished. At the end of her essay on page 50, she admits the attrition model isn't the only one, and invites people to develop their own by saying, "we need a plethora of workable models." In the primary model presented in this book, the meaning model, the process is by "crowding out" what isn't meaningful with what is. It starts with crowding out as much as we can of sick, disease, disabled, and ill from our consciousness. Crowding out is by re-uncovering the meaning we discovered in mania that was ignored via gaslighting. Since we have limited bandwidth, adding our meaning will eventually push the medical model out of our consciousness, except for practical purposes. We don't need to identify as mentally ill to utilize whatever we need from the medical model. We don't need to identify with an apple to eat it. We can shift our orientation to the meaning model. *Psychiatry Disrupted* goes as far as to say that we "tacitly acknowledge the authority of psychiatry by the sheer act of appealing to it." That's why we are going to crowd it out by the end of this book.

Neuroscientist Dr. Daniel Siegel says that "integration is differentiation and then linkage" and "mind is energy and information flow."[39] By processing our experiences for ourselves, we integrate and make up our minds. Mind can make mind. Our mind is energy and information flow. By changing our energy and information flow, we are changing and creating our minds. Our energy and information flow, or mind, has been ready-made for all of us. By endeavoring in this game, we are doing fundamental work in human consciousness. Processing our own experiences is a human necessity. We differentiate our experiences from the medical model and link them to our other models to build a new web of meaning.

But I'm not done with *Psychiatry Disrupted* yet. On page 178, Rosemary Barnes and Susan Schellenberg point out the importance of "individuals with lived experience naming and responding in and on [their] own terms rather than deferring to the constructs specified by mental health professionals" and the need to "displace the medical model as the dominant social narrative for naming and responding to emotional pain."[4] This is the game-changer. We don't need to find meaning; we need to create it. We don't need to seek the narrative; we need to create it. We need more narratives based on infinite possibilities, meaning, inner explorations, and superpowers—not only pain. We need to put what our experiences mean where they can be seen and not leave them buried, mistranslated, and locked away in psychiatrists' notes.

We need to consciously shed limiting inner language structures. Language is behavior, and as it is, language is behaving badly in our mind space. Our voice is the biggest and most underutilized tool. Your being is a director and creator of meaning. We are developing a voice of our own beyond being a parrot. When we make meaning, we make sense, or sense the meaning crafted in our consciousness. However we choose to make sense of our experiences, it doesn't have to make sense in all contexts. It can be transient or fleeting. It can make sense at the moment that it made sense in, and that's it. We are allowed to make sense to and for ourselves in any given moment. Psychiatry says we don't have permission to think, see, feel, and do in certain ways. Of course, we never want to harm ourselves or others. That would happen less if we didn't fear our experiences, creating a vicious cycle of fear that can lead to chaos, confusion, and harm. Whether we are on the spectrum of recovery, antipsychiatry, or are a consumer-survivor, we need to join together.

SOME WORDS ON SUFFERING AND GROWTH

"Most human suffering stems from tension created by the difference between the actual and potential self. This duality also reveals itself as manifested vs. un-manifested, real vs. imaginary, and body vs. spirit. Mind is the complex operator that resolves the difference between these opposites, and "assembles" them together into manifested reality. The problems that arise in life do so to help resolve this tension."

- Don Estes

Identity Politics

It's not taboo to talk about the suffering involved in bipolar 'disorder.' We've become courageous enough to share the suffering we go through. We are allowed to make the suffering part into something real, even though others can't see or feel the pain we do. We are allowed to make an identity out of suffering. We need to stop shaming each other for talking about the positives and making them real, even though others can't see it. I'd rather have chronic positivity than chronic suffering. It could be beneficial, and we won't know unless we give it a fair try. Maybe it matters what we give our attention to. If we talk about the positive half as much as we talk about the negatives, we could tip the energetic scales, and who knows what could happen. We would ask for support with the positives of bipolar as well as the negatives since we are experiencing both. Here's an example of a response to one of my tweets that illustrates strong identification with the negatives and suffering:

> Me: "It's empowering to re-language [bipolar] for some because they don't experience it as a disorder? Like bipolarity, bipolarism, omnipolar (all directions), bipolar spectrum, bipolar spiritism, bipolar diverse-order, bipolar, or of course bipolar disorder."

> Reply: "bipolar spiritism? Gosh {this} identity politics is a bit over the top. It is diagnosed as a disorder when there is impairment and disability. All these identity types are taking the piss and can f#ck off. Minimizing the struggles of those with diagnosed disorders."

> Me: "It depends what part we want to identify with. We

are taught to identify with the worst parts and neglect to think about the "abilitation" and renewal that happens at times too. It's taboo to talk about the positives. I don't want to minimize the good things bipolar has brought."

Reply: "it's both in my experience. There are some benefits from bipolar and there are some trade-offs. Can be times of accomplishments and times of suffering."

This person gifted me the perspective of identity politics. I'd never thought about it that way. Bipolar disorder includes identity politics. Disorder only works if we take it on, identify with it, make it part of our identity and then defend it like it's part of who we are. But that's not the problem. Why do we so strongly identify with the suffering side of the spectrum and forget about the positives? Why do we give suffering more staying power than it already has? Why do we spread negativity about the suffering and rarely spread positivity about the enlightening aspects? We are hypervigilant for negative "triggers." Is there an equal and opposite word that we can identify with for the positives, like perhaps "sparkers?" Imagine if we endeavored to talk about our sparkers as much as our triggers?

Suffering Attached to Beingness

We are so attached to suffering, we end up playing the victim instead of visionary. We forget our visionary nature. We neglect to share positive possibilities and memes. We end up believing we are less than rather than remembering we have more to offer. I'm not talking about pretending away the suffering. I'm asking: why don't we lean into putting a bit more, or equal attention on the visionary side of the bipolar spectrum and see what happens.

Don't worry, we're going to go into it together. Why is suffering the default and joy so challenging to muster? We need to defend our ecstasy, not physically, but in a type of thesis defense. The narratives from mental illness literature have become our groupthink. This, after discovering so deeply we have a mind and life of our own imbued with great power. If you didn't have a bipolar diagnosis, you might be reading something similar in a book in the genre of metaphysics or new age stuff, hoping to raise your vibration. So, it's totally fine for us bipolar people to explore the same vibration of information to help us make sense of our experiences after the fact. It's the same process but in reverse.

When we live outside the box in dimensions of life that are ecstatic, the return to the box is painful instead of normal. Suffering takes us over and lives our life for us. We suffer for reasons too complex to go into and the topic of many other books. In simple terms, the mainstream life we bought into without consent is Maya, or illusion, and believing in it is suffering. After mania, we can sink into the suffering state of depression, with or without a trip through psychosis. Despite this, there are still good aspects of being and having bipolar. We don't focus on the good parts of mania or bipolar, even though there is nothing stopping us but the taboo. We are told it'll make it worse. Really, if they admitted that going into it would be helpful, they'd have to provide support like counseling to do so, and they just don't have the resources. I was saddened by an Instagram post where a woman shared that she didn't share for 20 years because she thought it would make her symptoms worse. Dr. Daniel Seigel said, "Where attention goes, neural firing flows, and neural connection grows."[40] In mania, we get to know the power of our attention and we need to use it. We go back into mania at some point despite the best treatments, so why not put our attention on its content before the next rollercoaster ride and prepare through integration? Wouldn't this strengthen the neural networks related to mania, and make it less intense? If there is more firing and more wiring, we have more strength for next time.

If we focus mainly on suffering, it brings up anxiety, fear, anger, grief, shame…all things that contribute to the suffering in bipolar disorder. There is a concept called "allostatic load" which means accumulation of the burden of stress.[41] The way we are told to see ourselves works against us as a vicious downward spiraling force. We need to keep stress low, as we are more susceptible to it. Focusing on the negatives and identifying with suffering increases stress and allostatic load. We have some work to do to tip the scales to put our attention on firing and wiring new neural networks. Also, by going into the positives, we can more accurately and clearly deal with the perceived disordered aspects with an open and curious mindset. Chronic stress and suffering distort whatever is happening now.

Life by Pathography or Post-Estasis Growth

A diagnosis puts a big part of our attention on the identity that there's something wrong with us. We adopt a pathography, which is defined as a "historical biography from a medical, psychological, and psychiatric standpoint."[42] Another definition of pathography is a "biography that focuses on a person's illness, misfortunes, or failures."[43] When diagnosed, we are implicitly handed maladaptive schemas like social isolation, defectiveness, dependance, failure, subjugation, and approval seeking. We somehow have to try to crawl out of this while sacrificing our own experience, pretending we trust in being enmeshed in an authoritative psychiatric paradigm. When asked to share our story, they expect to hear our pathography and our journey to try to be sufficient in a world of illusory standards.

What if we also have an ecstasography? What if we have a collection of our visions, fortunes, gifts, and successes that came from bipolar mania? Yes, I have bipolar disorder. I'm also a self-identified mystic, philosopher, and Bodhisattva. What if we told our ecstasography as well or instead? Besides, it's closer to the truth we want to live out. We have to speak it into existence. Over the years of sharing my story with family members supporting their loved ones with mental illness, I've transitioned to share my ecstasography. Over time we need to say it to normal people so we can build bridges to show normal is not the only valid reality. When they don't project shame, fear, and confusion onto their loved ones, and fill the house with that energy, a different relationship is possible.

We can create and try different perspectives, so we don't default to our pathography. Can we create branches of wisdom and possibilities that lead to human potential and our wildest dreams? We need more choices and options in how we make sense of our experiences and how we understand ourselves internally, as well as the practical. We are going to use our lived expertise on a new level. You may have heard that trauma can lead to growth. According to a Wikipedia page, there is a positive side to trauma or crisis:

> *Posttraumatic growth or benefit finding is positive psychological change experienced as a result of adversity and other*

challenges in order to rise to a higher level of functioning. These circumstances represent significant challenges to the adaptive resources of the individual, and pose significant challenges to their way of understanding the world and their place in it.[44]

Trauma is a part of bipolar, whether from childhood or the psychiatric system itself. We can experience posttraumatic growth, whether we know about the concept or not. Along the same lines, can we experience what I call "Postecstasis Growth," or positive psychological change resulting from the ecstasy in mania? Can we use mania to rise to a higher level of functioning in the areas that mania augments? Ecstasy is challenging, and it's framed as negative or traumatic by the illness system. It is traumatic to see there is a level so elevated, alive, and vibrant that it makes all of life before it seems totally violent and nonsensical. Then, going back to the normal world feels traumatic like a waking nightmare. In normal life, we live in a matrix of trauma, and we don't notice until we poke our head above it. When we are dunked back into the matrix, we're gasping with fear.

It's a well-established fact people diagnosed with mental illness have more adverse childhood experiences and/or recent traumatic events. Count me in that category. Despite this, pills come before psychotherapy because it's easier to sweep issues under the 'drug.' The out-of-control ups and downs of bipolar can be traumatic in themselves. The content in bipolar experiences can be traumatic. Going to the psych ward is traumatic. Trying to recover within the psychiatric and recovery framework is traumatic. Do we go from mania to depression? Or do we go from mania to oppression? What about bipolar growth–the growth we undergo via mutating from normal consciousness to bipolar consciousness? The book *Waking the Tiger: Healing Trauma* by Peter Levine says that trauma is one of the pathways to enlightenment.[45] This means we can utilize our trauma as a pathway to enlightenment if we look at it that way.

Though we may still feel like victims of mental illness, a victim mentality doesn't help us. I remember experiencing a therapy with a naturopath where he made statements about a recent trauma, and I then could respond. It also involved feedback from my body. At one point he said, "and we're going to fight this." I immediately burst out crying and kept repeating, "I don't want to fight! I don't want to fight." When I left, I felt determined to do more good than fighting how I'd been harmed. I wanted to focus on the good that I could do rather than fighting being victimized. I didn't want to play victim. I didn't want to fight. Was it the right decision? I don't know, but I felt it so strongly I could do nothing else. Six months later I went manic, then psychotic, then to the psych ward. By trying to be strong and taking it on myself, my trauma turned into my personal brain illness. Maybe I should have stood up for myself then, but I wouldn't change this bipolar diagnosis because it's given me so many gifts. Without bipolar, I might have remained a victim. I tried my best to go into goodness, and I went into mania. Mania showed me my power, and I know I'm not a victim when I'm in my power. Power should not be used to profit from vulnerable people. That's not real power. I'm interested in what is present when we befriend the darkness and talk about what we experience when we rise above it. Can mania and psychosis be transformed from a vicious to a virtuous cycle?

FROM RECOVERY TO UN-RECOVERY TO RE-UNCOVERY

"Most individuals fearing, the complex depths within, remain at the superficial and surface layers of their psyche."

- Friedrich Nietzsche

The New Recovery Approach is Already Outdated

The latest approach in the mental health system is called the recovery approach. Despite its buzz and novelty, the recovery movement is already outdated. Consider how we were institutionalized for life not too long ago—the ice baths, insulin comas, and lobotomies. There was little belief in recovery from the practitioners. Most of us didn't recover because the system's approach thought we couldn't. Now the mental health system says we can recover and live in the community[46], and poof, we do. So, what else can we do? How long are we going to wait for the system to tell us what the next movement is? If we do, it can only be a modified extension of paternalism. How long do we wait for their slow research and evidence-based practices to tell us what we can do next? If we do, we will be twenty years older and not any wiser. How long do we wait for them to apply human potential frameworks, leading-edge information, and science outside of psychiatry to people with mental illnesses? It's our turn to decide what we can do next! We can't stop giving ourselves a memetic lobotomy by thinking what we've been told to think and start thinking for ourselves. We can look at ourselves however we want and create ourselves however we choose, regardless of how we are gazed at and treated by the system.

Waiting for evidence-based practices is too slow. Researchers study drugs and treatments for years, then it takes years for that evidence to become an evidence-based practice. It takes years for it to be adopted into practice on a wide scale. By that time, that best practice is already waiting to be replaced by the next one, and on and on. Meanwhile, many of us live unfulfilled lives and die 9-25 years before our undiagnosed bretheren.[47] We must create the quantum leap we need to remove ourselves from this prison and early death trap.

No wonder I've never liked the word recovery. It's already condemned and loaded. A "recovery mission" is to retrieve a dead body. Is a recovery movement to make me into a dead man walking? To me, recovery implies that mainstream reality is the only reality, and we must adjust back into a reality that is dying, and thus feel deadened. It's a dead end. We are deficient and need to return to our old way of being, even though it wasn't working. Recovery implies that we should endeavor to ignore anything that was positive in mania. We are never encouraged or supported to go over what happened in mania and form meaning from it. We need integration and transformation, not just recovery. Recovery attempts to "re-cover" over the problems and keep them hidden and suppressed, but not healed, with medications and treatments. We also re-cover over the positive aspects of mania—visions, information, insights, and ideas. We are told what we experienced wasn't real and that we need to recover back into what is real. Why then does mania feel more real? We feel more real to ourselves—like the "real me," though others don't like it. Reality feels more real when I'm me. We feel true to who we are and what's happening now, rather than a cog in society's machinery and programming. Recovery is to force us back into being a cog in society's machinery, disregarding any new ways we wish to explore living our lives.

Empowered People Are Dangerous to the Status Quo

An empowered human has a great effect on consciousness, whether they sit in a cave or make a piece of toast. The quality of human consciousness is more important than the quantity of menial work. We need more qualitative aspects in human beings to emerge because of the over-emphasis on the quantitative. We are told to "re-cover" from our delusional experience in favor of working at Starbucks for a few hours a week. When we wake up from a dream, we realize it was just a dream, and we soon forget what it was about because it wasn't real. When we come back from mania, we never forget how mania felt more real than this world. We never forget our insights and profound experiences, even if they get buried under tranquilizers or we have the sh*t shocked out of us. Manic consciousness is a state I call "super-awake." Once we've been super-awake, regular wakefulness feels like living in the Matrix. The Matrix is a metaphor for the reality of two distinct worlds. One is the usual state we call awake, and the other is the super-awake state of real wakefulness. People don't seem alive or real when in mania because we are super-awake. We can get irritated when others aren't as energetic or euphoric. Mania can lead to the experience of the zombie apocalypse because sometimes sleepwalkers seem zombie-like. We are forced to come back, smile and nod, and nod off into the consensus world, until we forget we didn't consent to it. We waste our life, for what?

J. Krishnamurti is attributed with saying, "It is no measure of health to be well-adjusted to a profoundly sick society."[48] It follows that it's no measure of health to recover back to being well-adjusted to a profoundly sick society. Recovery implies that the whole problem lies within the individual. In his book City Shadows Arnold Mindell states "Someone with unusual mental experiences, someone in an 'extreme state' is not just ill, but a 'city shadow', a part of our larger collective, a voice that is usually marginalized as insignificant."[49] Not only are we more sensitive, but we can also pick up on unprocessed energies that others ignore. Somebody has to pay for it. It's like holographic trash that someone else must pick up. Suffering has to go somewhere and gets transferred to others. Think about when someone has a traumatic experience and is fully supported by family, friends, and practitioners. Some of the suffering goes to others, but they are appropriately reacting in a timely fashion to disperse the trauma. If someone experiences trauma but there is no appropriate help at the right time, all that energy is still there, emanating from the person to other people. All sorts of drama and violence can play out because of the lack of love. More suffering and trauma are accumulated because others wield their power when they see vulnerable people. We don't know how to recognize trauma, and we don't take responsibility. The madness is all of ours, and it's all of our responsibility, not just those with a label. We are the scapegoats and the canaries in the coal mine. We get crucified.

Re-Uncovery or UnRecovered

There are many reasons why, rather than thinking in terms of recovery, I prefer to see the process as re-uncovery—an opportunity to rediscover, redesign and re-create life anew, now. I came across a website Recovery in the Bin,[6] that also criticized the term recovery. They created a term "unrecovery." Here are some points from their website:

What we believe:

1 – *We believe that the concept of 'recovery' has been co-opted by mental health services, commissioners, and policy makers.*

2 – *We believe the growing development of this form of the 'Recovery Model' is a symptom of neoliberalism, and that capitalism is at the root of the crisis! Many of us will never be able to 'recover' living under these intolerable social and economic conditions, due to the effects of circumstances such as poor housing, poverty, stigma, racism, sexism, unreasonable work expectations, and countless other barriers.*

3 – *We believe that the term 'UnRecovered' is a valid and legitimate political self-definition (not a permanent description of anyone's mental state) and we emphasise its political and social contrast to 'Recovered.' This doesn't mean we want to remain 'unwell' or 'ill' but that we reject the new neoliberal intrusion on the word 'recovery' that has been redefined, and taken over by market forces, humiliating treatment techniques, and homogenising outcome measurements.*

I recommend reading their website for more on how they address the politics of recovery. We are going to continue with potential and possibilities. I'm hoping to crowd out much of what I'm saying now as we go along. This includes putting attention on venting about the mental health system to juxtapose it to re-uncovery. What mania points to doesn't need juxtaposition to the mental health system at all. Just look at human potential, metaphysical, and spiritual perspectives on growth. Mania is the same heightened energy bestowed non-volitionally, surprisingly, instead of being consciously earned through intentional study and practice. Mania is about un-limitation too, and we need to build bridges to new expansive territory. To build a bridge, we must start from where we are. The mental health system is about limitations. Until then, it seems the system seeks to 'unmagic' mania and I am pro-manic magic. Rather than being in opposition to the old, we will be in juxtaposition. Our new positions will crowd out the old to an appropriate small proportion of the possibilities. Recovery in the Bin also states, "We reserve the right to ridicule and satirise what we dislike rather than always respond with reasoned arguments which can get a bit boring and bad for our mental health."[50] In the context of manic magic, I'd say we reserve the right to focus on the light of mania's human potential. We reserve the right to respond with metaphors, extrapolations, meaning, magic, energy, silence, space, neologisms, riffs, rhymes, the invisible, context, gesture, synchronicity, song, insights, manic information, lived experience, etc...

False Security in Recovery

Despite the best efforts of the recovery movement, 4-19% of bipolar people still die by suicide.[7] There is a danger that lies in the meaninglessness of being disempowered. Meaninglessness leads to hopelessness, and hopelessness can lead to suicide. Bipolar can be dangerous if unmanaged, but it can be equally dangerous if 'un-magicked.' Medications are a key factor in the un-magicking process. Medications keep us within certain limits and turn down the volume on the non-ordinary to help us do practical things. They tranquilize the brain and inhibit learning and growing. We feel tired, sluggish, knocked out, clumsy, unmotivated, and unable to concentrate or think. These things are blamed on the illness, even though there are few studies of unmedicated people with a diagnosis.

Studies have shown antipsychotics decrease brain volume and that long-term medication maintenance treatment has failed to produce good outcomes.[51] The word "outcome" really grinds my gears. We aren't outcomes. Like anyone else, we are humans with lives that mean something. If you are someone on antipsychotics and your brain is shrinking, you aren't thinking about good outcomes. I'm one of the lucky ones who benefits from medications, though I'd like not to be on four of them, including an antipsychotic. In Finland, they also use the Open Dialogue approach and have put a new lens on psychosis and schizophrenia. They are now beginning to study this approach in the USA. Why don't they use the Finnish studies success and start providing Open Dialogue now? Is American's psychosis that different from Finnish psychosis? In Finland through Open Dialogue, something like two-thirds of people who go into psychosis get back to the workforce in two years. Only 10-15% of people labeled with schizophrenia return to work under the current recovery model[52], not that returning to a mediocre job is exciting or a true sign of one's humanity.

We must recover practical tasks like personal hygiene, preparing meals, and dressing ourselves. We also need to "re-uncover" what we uncovered in mania, that got covered back up by diagnosis. Otherwise, we can fall victim to a lack of personal meaning. We went into mania to see that meaning is everywhere, and especially to give us hope beyond trauma. We return to the state of meaninglessness and trauma. We need look back and harvest our meanings to compensate; to get some benefit out of the cost of being traumatized and returning to trauma. We can build a bridge between the meaningless world and the meaningful world that is our nature. This is different than "recovery" and being "unrecovered" above. Each time we re-uncover something, we can integrate it. If our brain thinks of something from a magical experience, it's re-uncovering. This way, what we uncovered can serve its purpose. Reverse metamorphosis back to the matrix is hard, but we do it. What do you wish to re-uncover?

WHAT'S IN THE WAY OF A NEURODIVERSITY PERSPECTIVE OF BIPOLAR?

"I am not the equivalent of my diagnosis.
The diagnosis is simply a set of words
used by someone to describe what they
think they see about me. I am free to
grow, to evolve, to reframe how I think and
experience myself. I need not be reduced
to the label that has been affixed to me."

– Mel Schwartz, The Possibility Principle[53]

I'm Not the Equivalent of My Diagnosis

The statement by Mel Schwartz reads like an affirmation. It's a challenge to be diagnosed bipolar and not be reduced to our affixed label. The label may help us fix some part of our life by accessing resources, but it doesn't fix everything. What's in the way? Maybe what we've accepted as "the way" is in fact "in the way."

I once attended a Hearing Voices Study Club group, and I was happily surprised by the group guidelines which included "making no assumption of illness."[54] Imagine if we were given the luxury of no assumption of illness while being involuntarily detained? Instead, the opposite assumption is true. We are guilty and there is no way to prove our innocence. If we don't accept that we have an illness, we lack insight into our illness–the aforementioned catch-22. This inability to be aware of an illness or as part of an illness is called "anosognosia."[55]

When I was diagnosed bipolar in the psych ward, the word bipolar was a bridge back to consensus reality. The experiences I had when I was "ill" with mania and psychosis, I experienced as real, rich, and spiritual, as well as confusing and terrifying. I knew there was no point in arguing with the doctor because I was being held involuntarily under the mental health act. Anything I said would be used to prove I was ill. They medicated me the moment I got there. I was already in the paradigm before they had time to give me a diagnosis. I was already made ill before I had time to prove that it was only temporary blip. I was guilty before I could prove my sanity. I was put on antipsychotic medications at maintenance treatment doses which distorted and addicted my brain function. I had insight into the catch-22 I found myself in. I had to submit to the narrative and treatment because I was already on it before I regained my senses after a few days. In order to earn the right to be allowed out of the hospital I had to somehow adapt to the foreign chemicals which, sadly and appropriately anchored me to a now foreign world.

Ironically, by pretending I was okay with the treatment by passively going along with it, I was becoming sane again. And many of us pretend we agree, or voice that we don't agree and get treated anyway. What are the other options? Fight and get restrained and injected? Or flee and get found and re-committed? Some of us go along with it because that's the only way to get access to the financial resources and other resources we need to survive in this disabling world. Still, it comes at a high social cost, side effects, and cumulative toxicity to the body organs. We don't get our blood tested because the medications are making us physically healthier. I've been taking lithium for 10 years and it's a not a matter of if, but when the drug will have done too much damage to my kidneys so that I must stop taking it. Bipolar might explain why I was back in the consensus world, but it didn't relate at all to the mysterious world I returned from, though it indicates I would likely return there in another mania. Expectations of release from the hospital included agreeing to recover back into the old ways and take medication. I decided to go along with it rather than resist it because of my agreement with the Universe to stay on Earth with my loved ones. It's easy to be angry in retrospect. At the same time, I see that it happened the way it happened as it happened that way. What's important to me is that I learned from it every step of the way.

It's Normal for the Brain to Resist

After mania, the brain resists going back to operating in the old world and fitting into a false culture. The false culture is reductionistic and material. The real world is expansionistic and ethereal. From our perspective, it's not because we're ill. Society's design is ill. It's designed so we live mechanistically, rather than being and creating ourselves anew. The default state that we live in is controlled by the default mode network in the brain. It's a categorically lower-energy state than mania and requires less of the brain and body's resources. Part of its mechanistic nature is to limit us to our habitual ways of acting. As such, our degrees of freedom of possibilities are limited to what the ego permits. Connecting with the present cannot happen through habit, requiring a higher energy state of the mind and body. It needs more energy to connect, but the connection creates greater energy than it needs once it's established. The brain is fueled by the novelty, spontaneity, and learning that connecting with the present moment facilitates. Mania is the activation energy required to connect to the present, or "what is." After that, our participation in the present moment catalyzes a positive feedback loop that yields more energy and information in a sustained way. Our default state wastes energy in repetition.

Even when mania is over, there's always a part of us that remains connected to the magic of the eternal moment. The "disability" or "disorder" is how society receives those who go into nonvolitional altered states. We get turned into the mental health system which turns us into mental patients. This is why some of us are surprised we are expected to think of ourselves as mentally ill. It's not from lack of insight into our illness, but profound insight into the nature of reality beyond the human-constructed world. The ego or our default mode of operation, has anosognosia as well. It has no insight into its programmed, mechanistic, and limited functioning. After mania, we understand, or at least our subconsciousness understands, the disability of going back to being our ego-self and its disabled nature—it can't go beyond its programming. That's why it's near impossible to "cure" our illness. The illness doesn't lie within us. We've seen another world and our brain tried to operate there without limitation. We lose our ability to be limited. And yet we can't maintain our unlimited aspect. Our ego-self was unaware of its illusions of living in a false reality that we thought was real. Now we know different. You can't put a butterfly back into a chrysalis. Yet society, which expects us to be a cog in the machinery of the economy, isn't designed for the abilities and spontaneity of those who shift into trans-conscious modes. Society works to actively suppresses Trans-Consciousness in favor of consistency and conformity.

I'm Not Crazy, You Are

The question of where the madness resides is nothing new. Here's another perspective from an excerpt from an episode titled "A True Madness – Schizophrenia" from the 1969 TV show called "Horizon":

> *Madness is not what happens to a person but what happens between people. Our behavior not only depends on what we want, but what other people expect. If schizophrenics live in disturbed families, they have to fit into false and rigid relationships. The sensitive finds this difficult. He has to live up to the role assigned him and suppress his own idea of himself. He can't contact those near him without being false to himself. schizophrenia is not Jekyll and Hyde, but false-self and real self. The mask is the false-self that the family needs. But behind is the real self-stunted and cut off. As he acts out his false-self, his family are happy because that's how they want him. He's being something that he isn't. Imprisoned in a closed family world his position is untenable. Going mad he asserts his real self.*

He says his family are trying to kill him, for example. Meaning in a poetic sense, they're not allowing him to be real. He's now refusing to play according to the family's rules in a game that's been destroying him. Once the rules have been challenged, the family can either examine the game that's disguising their own problems or call him mad. Threatened with a reappraisal of their own life, it's easier to choose the latter.[56]

Though this is an old perspective, acting out a false version of ourselves to play a part others want is still seen as normal today. An unnamed French writer and lecturer Jean-Ives Leloup coined the term "normosis" meaning a "pathology of normality, characterized by conformity and adaptation, in large scale, to a morbid context."[57] Happily, bipolar and normosis are mutually exclusive terms and experiences. I'd rather be maladjusted to a crazy possible reality than well-adjusted to one that's going extinct. If the old normal wasn't normosis already, the new normal is surely a morbid, largescale context that we are forced to adapt to. I once read how hugs boost the immune system, maybe more than any medical intervention.[58] We need upwards of twelve per day. Being deprived of human touch and oxytocin has untold consequences for us and future generations. The three main things that increase blood circulation are sunshine, grounding or touching our skin to the Earth, and human touch. If our blood doesn't circulate optimally, our cells are deprived of oxygen, and they die. Additionally, fear suppresses the immune system. Most of us know this in theory. But we aren't afraid of what being afraid does to our immune system enough to stop being afraid–another catch-22. We have anosognosia of what fear does to us. Maybe we should fear the normosis of being afraid.

In an article titled "The Danger of 'Normosis'," Paulo Roberto R. Ferriera said:

> *Normal people are the most dangerous "thing." Normal People created this sick society and lead the planet to the current destruction state. We will need many, many "crazy" ones to fix everything...Normal is, by definition, something that corresponds to a norm. How could such diverse creatures as humans be "fitted" to norm, as in a mold? If it fits, something will be ignored and left out of the mold...parts will be missing...or neurosis will be overflowing.[59]*

Psychoanalyst Joyce McDougall coined the term "normopathy" which means "the pathological pursuit of conformity and societal acceptance at the expense of individuality."[60] From the lived experience perspective, the recovery movement could also be called normopathy. We try to fit in at the expense of our individuality. She says, "Normopathy is difficult to diagnose because normopaths are integrated in society. Normopaths depend on social approval and validation."[60] In mania, the fact that we don't need validation, follow social norms, or need social approval is a sign of illness. Aldous Huxley speaks to the sadness of the pathology of normality:

> *"The real hopeless victims of mental illness are to be found among those who appear to be most normal. Many of them are normal because they are so well adjusted to our mode of existence, because their human voice has been silenced so early in their lives that they do not even struggle or suffer or develop symptoms as the neurotic does. They are normal not in what may be called the absolute sense of the word; they are normal only in relation to a profoundly abnormal society. Their perfect adjustment to that abnormal society is a measure*

of their mental sickness. These millions of abnormally normal people, living without fuss in a society to which, if they were fully human beings, they ought not to be adjusted."[61]

Moving Away from Normal

Normal seems to mean afraid, obedient, programmable, controllable, susceptible to marketing, media, and Pavlovian conditioning. Fortunately, there are many peers and movements working diligently to correct the pathology of normality. If you've been called bipolar, you've been doing your part by going into uncharted inner and outer territories, whether you've been aware of the significance of it or not. It's important that someone explore as nonvolitional pyschonauts or we'd have all been doomed to be normopaths long ago. Society has anosognosia of the importance of psychonauts who can journey outside the norm by whatever means. Otherwise, we are doomed as humanoid robots, or worse. Indigenous Peoples often go into a trance and don't base their decisions on the material world. We should have been respecting, revering, and collaborating with the Indigenous Peoples all along. We wouldn't be in the mess we're in. Perhaps we suffer from mental illness because we lack the wisdom from the First Nations and the Peoples who are in relationship with the land. Hopefully de-colonization includes colonizing the western mind with the suppressed wisdom and nature-mysticism through deep listening and dialogue— to transfer and absorb the truths in our genome and meme pool. Other non-western cultures have wisdom traditions and have less mental illness and more healing when they don't use Western methods. The western world doesn't recognize wisdom traditions and other ways of accessing information. In mania, we act and behave on our inner subjective meaning, but we don't have a wisdom tradition to back it up and make sense of it. This vulnerability makes us easy to be converted to mental patients. On the creative maladjustment week website, they invite what they call "healers from normal":

> MindFreedom International is working along with "the real" psychiatric survivor/physician/clown, PATCH ADAMS to invite everyone who is a "healer of normal"! ...Rev. Martin Luther King, Jr. repeatedly said – for more than a decade – that he was proud to be what psychologists called "maladjusted" because, "The salvation of the world lies in the hands of the creatively maladjusted."[62]

Are we maladjusted to a profoundly sick society, or are we adjusting to a transformed consciousness and a transformed world, leaving the sick world behind? People called mentally ill sometimes exhibit "apophenia," or the tendency to spot patterns where none exist.[63] We are told the patterns, relationships, and connections we make aren't real. But what about the opposite. "Randomania" means "attributing chance probability to (apparently) related phenomenon (specifically in contrast to apophenia)."[64] Maybe there is too much randomania in the minds of those suffering from normosis? We need to see new patterns of oneness over the prevailing chaos of division and destruction. It's crazy not to see the meanings in the interrelatedness and interconnectedness of things or be aware of something new in the moment. We create the meaningful patterns, not just passively observe them. The meaning could be up to us. But it's normal to ask the authorities for social approval about what is the meaning of life. The inner conflict between who we are and who we should be is the source of the chaos and violence in the world. As a result of the tension, we don't know who we are and can't do what we don't know we should otherwise be doing. Our life is meaningless.

Much Too Much Heaven on Earth

What if we didn't have to end up going mad to resolve the conflict? Where would we be, and what would society look like if we were all who we are as the rule and not the exception? Heaven on Earth much? If life were designed to maintain our original alignment with the source of ourselves from day one, what would this world and society look like? Harmonious, ingenious, beautifully stewarded, bathed in a light of golden-green. But how do we correct the misalignment from ourselves when it's been going the wrong direction on for so long? How do you move a globe from one track to another? That's where mania comes in. It restores us to our original trajectory and source. If people who go into mania integrated their embodiment, it would make it easier for others. Multiple worlds exist and we leap through many parallel worlds to get to the world we originated for ourselves. Michael Jackson said, "And the dream we were conceived in will shine again in grace."

If we grew up this way, we wouldn't need a super energetic mania to correct the cognitive dissonance of living in a default mode. Mania is an emergency response from the nervous system to meaninglessness. Our possibilities still exist folded up in the present, and mania unfolds them in an instant so we can find instant meaning. We can radically shape shift and speed up to access other possibilities. We make others uncomfortable because we are operating outside the game of theory of mind, norms, and so we aren't predictable. Predictability is needed to be controlled. We can't be controlled unless we are medicated. We challenge the tradition that personal change only happens slowly and progressively. We challenge the myth that we can't make up for lost time and be who we are now. It's never too late. More and more of us will find our star quality later in life until the gap closes, and we never lose ourselves in the first place. The world needs each of us to come alive. We won't sacrifice our individuality and accept this normosis. Psychosis is the scary journey back to normosis.

Cookie Cutter Crazy

Part of coming alive is diversity of perception, experience, language, and gifts. Society assumes everyone should fit into a cookie-cutter mold. If we don't, we risk having the diversity tranquilized out of us. Increasingly more kids are being medicated so they can sit in a chair in a classroom for six hours a day and "learn." If they can't do this, they are defective because aren't fitting in as a cog in the machine of society. Kids are lab rats moving towards the rat race. All the while, anyone with a brain could be the next person strapped into a straitjacket and diagnosed with a serious and persistent mental illness for life. It was me, so it could be you or anyone you care about.

We get pulled down from the rapture of mania and get captured. I like the term "experience police," which I read in the book "The Politics of Experience" by R.D. Laing.[65] Do we have bipolar disorder or is our experience is subjected to "experience-ism?" Similarly, denying the reality of another's subjective perception and experience could be called "perception-ism" as well as gaslighting. It's denying the truth of the capacity of subjectivity to create meaning that is displayed on the mindscreen as perception. When we subject someone to perception-ism or experience-ism, we are burning their book. Meaningful events in our lives get systematized and explained away as just an illness with no meaning. This could be called "meaning-ism." We can go as far as to create "consciousness-ism" for disallowing diversity in consciousness and Trans-Consciousness. There is a bias towards what's thought to be normal consciousness. Neurodiveristy calls for a broader spectrum of included perceptions, meanings, subjectivity, personalities, and experiences without being drugged and denied full citizenship. We need diversity in consciousness to survive as a species, especially as we take up a greater percentage of the overall biomass.

Am I Un-Understanable So Far?

Are mental illness labels seen as necessary to explain otherwise "un-understandable" experiences? The term un-understandable was used by Karl Jaspers. A paper by Samei Huda, elaborates on what Jaspers implies:

> Jaspers explains "primary delusions" of schizophrenia as the observed manifestation of a global change in awareness of the world with altered meanings of experiences. In "delusions proper" there is a core to the underlying experience that is not accessible to others understanding as they do not share this changed awareness of the world. Jaspers describes this phenomenon as a qualitative change from normal or everyday experience that cannot be understood due to lack of shared meanings.[66]

Let's juxtapose that with another statement by Huda:

> *The strong psychological psychosis model states that for all the speech, gestures, behavior etc. labeled as functional psychosis we can show how they came about purely in terms of psychological events in a social context in the same way as anxiety or shyness, are continuous with normal psychological processes i.e., are not qualitatively different states and that the meaning of what is communicated can also be understood.*[66]

I share these two excerpts from the same paper to address some other points. In the first paragraph, Jaspers is correct in saying there is a changed awareness of the world and that it's a qualitative change from a lived experience perspective. The lazy way out is saying it's un-understandable or cannot be understood. The way to understand is through genuine listening and dialogue. The goal of psychiatry is to change the patient back to normal, not to listen. It's not to develop new understandings of a qualitatively changed awareness that is accessing a different part of reality.

The second paragraph takes the stance that normal and psychosis states aren't qualitatively different and that they are understandable. This adds insult to injury because, from a lived experience perspective, altered states are qualitatively different *and* understandable, which neither of the excerpts allows for. The paper says that if the experiences aren't qualitatively different, they are understandable; if they are qualitatively different, they are un-understandable. With the possibility of a qualitatively different state of awareness that is understandable, the only option is to engage in a dialogue to understand that state of awareness and its content and context. Both perspectives try to understand through listening to someone who has a diagnosis of schizophrenia. In both cases, they aren't trying to understand anything but confirming their paradigm.

The system still hasn't tried to understand lived experience. It doesn't matter much because we don't need our experiences to be understood by anyone but us. We don't have to remain un-understandable to ourselves. We can support others to understand the manic state we go into and do so on our own terms once we've integrated. Then we will create something similar to a dream interpretation book full of missing manic memes and meanings as a guide for others. Are we suffering from a mental illness or is there widespread anosognosia of normosis, normopathy, randomania, and conscious biases like experiencism, perceptionism, meaningism, consciousnessism and other "ism" patterns? Still, let's reframe and word the idea of spreading non-pathological ideas into positive terms. We are spreading positive, potential, meaningful, and magical ideas about bipolar, mania, psychosis, and Trans-Consciousness and other possible and parallel worlds, realities, and dimensions.

Digging a Hole of Defect

Another article emphasizes the unacknowledged harm of the illness lens. A clinical psychologist named Noel Hunter wrote an article called "Rising Rates of Suicide: When Do We Acknowledge that Something Isn't Working!?" What follows is an excerpt from his piece:

> *Telling a person they are "ill" for suffering or being sad serves to further alienate the individual. It often results in the person feeling defective, and puts the problem inside the individual*

instead of recognizing that cultural and circumstantial factors are a problem. Studies have demonstrated over and over again that a biological illness perspective on human suffering leads to decreased empathy, increased desire for social distance, and increased prejudice and discrimination...

In other words: we, as a society, are being told that if someone is suffering, the correct approach is to convince them of ideas that will likely lead them to feel marginalized, helpless, hopeless, worse about themselves, ashamed, retraumatized and less likely to reach out to others for connection and support when, in fact, connection and support are the very things most likely to heal. Logic at its finest.[67]

In addition to being ashamed and marginalized, the purely biological model makes us alienated and mistrusting of our own minds and bodies. We become an enemy of ourselves and this is a no win game. This division is an illusion. By now we can recognize the downside of emphasizing that perspective.

As much as we get called back to recover in the old paradigm world, we need to call forth the new paradigm. We need to have activities in both worlds, to learn to walk in and between them. We can be a guiding light for people adjusting to a profoundly magical, spontaneous, synchronous, and creative world. After all, people do all manners of things and take all kinds of substances to get out of the mundane mind. We are frequency holders to another world, anchored in this world by tranquillizing medications. It matters from where you look and what eyes you have to see. Then we see, we aren't objects to be subjected to society, and what we are is in and not of that world. What is it going to be? I think we'd both rather be magical, so let's light the way.

Part
TWO

Towards the Future-Present
Approach of Meaning

"We are here to find that
dimension within ourselves that is
deeper than thought."

- Eckhart Tolle

Chapter 3

WHEN YOU CHANGE THE WAY YOU LOOK AT THINGS…

THE DISCOVERY THAT OTHERS SEE IT TOO – I'M NOT ALONE IN THINKING OUTSIDE THE BIPOLAR BOX

"Every moment is a fresh new beginning, a wonderful inauguration of the great cosmic journey through the Universe. We can do whatever we want. We can change reality at any moment."

- Russell Brand

Lacking Insight into Our Illness Together

Dr. Wayne Dyer said, "When you change the way you look at things, the things you look at change." Mania changes the way we look at things, things change, and we behave different accordingly. The first time I discovered that

I wasn't alone in interpreting my experiences as meaningful was in the book *The Spiritual Gift of Madness* by Seth Farber. After nearly four years of thinking I was the only one who thought in alternative ways, and keeping it to myself, I was validated by how much I resonated with every word of Farber's book. His exposition affirmed everything I felt to be true in my heart. How did he know? I knew my experiences were valid, not delusion. I found two more books with overlapping themes, namely, *Rethinking Madness: Towards a Paradigm Shift in Our Understanding and Treatment of Psychosis* by Paris Williams and *Recovering Sanity: A Compassionate Approach to Understanding and Treating Psychosis* by Edward Podvoll. All three are very good reads.

More recently, I took a course on Udemy by Ron Unger called "Spiritual Issues Within Treatment for Psychosis and Bipolar." He is one of the few professionals I've found whose lectures and trainings for clinicians challenges the status quo thinking. His courses point out the possibility and importance of engaging psychosis to make sense of it. He presents a framework for seeing value in psychosis and bipolar. His thinking aligns with the themes of this book. I had to come to these same realizations myself through my exploration of my experience, so I was overjoyed to find Ron Unger's work. Here are a few points he makes in his course that are music to my ears:

- *It's not so much the experiences themselves but what people make of the experience that determines whether the experience contributes to someone's growth or not.*

- *And what people make of their experience is affected by the context they're in. Like how others react. This affects if experiences can be integrated into the rest of their life.*

- *Framing people's experience as nothing but an illness can be part of what impairs people's ability to relate to themselves or their experience. It becomes a self-fulfilling prophecy.*

- *If they can't find anything of value in it, they might miss out on a very important opportunity for growth.*

- *Something could still be a part of a person's process even if dark and negative.*

- *Sort through it successfully for the benefit of themselves and everyone.[35]*

I can't help but wonder what it might have been like to have a clinician with this background. For more genius from Ron Unger, I highly recommend his courses listed at recoveryfromschizophrenia.org/store. Unfortunately, the mental illness system, as it is currently, thinks that there is no point in trying to make sense of bipolar or psychotic experiences. The current approach prevents any possibility of integrating the experiences. They are repressed and resisted by being explained away as illness. Going into it is thought to stir the pot, humor the illusions, and make things worse. In my experience, these propositions are myths and don't hold up. We may be afraid to make sense of our experiences because we've been programmed to fear it. That is a disservice because it keeps us in a trap. Using my brain to learn about my experiences and what they could mean about life keeps my brain strong and growing. It keeps my brain in the field of meaning. When I make sense of my experiences for myself, it's less scary when a future psychosis happens. We can build a psychological immune system to neutralize fear. It's a bit like if someone studies martial arts, they are less afraid of being confronted with a fight. We have been impaired in our ability to relate to ourselves and our experiences because we haven't been encouraged to create and look through other frames other than illness.

Could I Love Me With All My Crazy?

I've endeavored to expand my understanding of my inner mindscape and experience, and I have the neural networks to go along with my efforts. By now, you may be wondering how you can do the same. We are getting there. I'm going to share what helped me understand so that I don't miss out on my dreams. Without it, I would have given up on my dreams and possibilities. When you begin to harvest your mania, opportunities for growth and purpose will emerge. Dark and negative aspects are also part of the process. If we can face the dark and the light, we can separate the signal in non-ordinary experiences from the noise to harvest the benefits.

The process eventually creates a web of meaning for new experiences to fall gently into in real-time. For now, we'll be integrating them intentionally with our conscious mind in retrospect. This is the re-uncovery process or meta-mania. The bigger the web of meaning we create, the more it can catch new experiences, and they won't be so energetic or jarring. While I was actively engaged in making sense and meaning out of my experiences, I had no hospitalizations in three years; yet I still went into crisis three times. I was plagued by three psych ward stays in fourteen months before I tried to understand. With my own self-expanded network and scaffolding of meaning, I was able to re-contextualize the events instead of escalating to a "fear of myself" response. My meaning created an "understanding of myself" response so I didn't spiral out of control. I'd made sense of chaos, so it was no longer chaos, but order. My order. I gained strength because it took a lot of strength to get through a crisis, even on the foundation I built. Engaging with my experiences via the process I created made things better, not worse. A simple example is realizing that a fearful thought doesn't mean I have to be afraid or act out the thought or react to it. It meant I stay present with the sensations in my entire body, and not create a division, where I run away from the intensity.

As we make sense, we create a vast web of meaning and context that can crowd out what is no longer helpful. Life becomes a process of our own making. Since it feels like we can create any life we want in mania, the activity of building meaning while not manic is in alignment with being 'a little bit manic all the time.' We are in essence being a bit manic without being manic. Then, we are more prepared for our next mania too. We enhance our own capacity to discover. In mania, we have so much going through our mind it has no space or time to integrate. When we look at it and consider it when we aren't manic, we give it space to integrate and associate in our mind. Then, when we do discover something if we are manic in the future, we have a context in our mind for it to be. This way, there is a smaller energetic gap between being in a state of mania and not being in mania, neurologically and memetically, because we've brought manic memes into our daily life, instead of resisting them. Often the same memes predominate during each cycle of mania, because they are suppressed and not given attention. When we give them attention, they will do what they need to do in our brains. We build an energetic mountain of our discoveries that builds a bridge between the two modes in Trans-Consciousness. The subjective experience of intensity, excitement, and overstimulation because our daily life has more flavors from mania. We've stimulated our brain with the stuff of mania daily to create a giant living puzzle. In my case, not engaging with my experience in mania and psychosis would have prevented the learning I needed to undertake. The system doesn't encourage this because they are not equipped with the time and tools to help us. The more we do this, we can create a wisdom tradition to support the next generation.

Traditionally Speaking

Some of the territory we encounter in mania has long been mapped by Eastern philosophy and tradition. Sciences such as physics and experiments in the human potential movement are groping at what the East has always known. Intellectual understanding is way behind lived experience too. Shamans, psychonauts, and the Indigenous Peoples could tell us more about what the West puts in the category of mental illness, if we listened. We might hear from them that the territory that the West calls mental illness has nothing to do with illness at all. The Brazilian Spiritists and their mental hospitals hold an alternative view. To them, mental disorders are caused by "suppressed mediumship." Emma Bragdon PhD says, "Brazilian Spiritists recognize those people who are gifted sensitives and in spiritual emergence and offer free training and help to stay in balance. Their paradigm of care has been cultivated since the 1860s."[68] From my understanding, they help people connect with their gifts because they've become mediums of the invisible realms and subtle domains. I resonate with being a medium of 'special messages' myself. Imagine if we were told, "You hear special messages? You must be a medium of special messages. We can support you with your mediumship."

It took me a bit of time to adapt to the special messages and to see that their specialness has nothing to do with me. Then I noticed the messages aren't that special. They are our natural birth rite, right from the source. The Universe can talk to any of us and pass along gifts and messages. A change in perception is needed to see it and be it. Our connection to the Universe cannot be broken. We are one with it. It feels special at first when we reconnect to the Universe after so long. Then we see the Universe is our constant companion.

Many mystics and gurus say humanity is sleepwalking, blind, and needs to wake up. Buddhism says what we consider reality is Maya, meaning "illusion." In mania, we discover the gurus are right. From our manic vantage point, we can see that the old paradigm is Maya, compared to the manic-nirvana world. Tranquilizers dampen "psi" phenomenon in favor of restoring functionality in the mainstream world. The authority of the mainstream narrative is pivotal. If we believe we are ill, we won't attempt to look at what is outside the scope of the medical paradigm. We won't realize our mediumship and connection with the Universe.

Other cultures recognize the same "symptoms" of mental illness as signs of possible initiation into training to become a Shaman. They understand that extra care, gentleness, unconditional love, and space are necessary for the individual to flower. The chaos is a good sign because it's a prerequisite to a breakthrough. The people know the signs for recognizing a potential Shaman, they are similar to signs of a mental health crisis. One day we'll be kept safe to integrate our healing journey without it being interrupted prematurely by tranquilizers. Each time a mania or psychosis happens, we'll be able to see how much we can integrate.

Good Luck for Bad Trips at Festivals

Though there is progress, systemic change is not happening fast enough to save those who are in need right now. The Zendo Project trains people to sit with those having a bad trip from taking psychedelics at festivals. If someone goes into a bad state, they are given a chance to get through it with the help of a supportive sitter, lessening the chance of getting carted away and put through a police intervention, followed by a trip to the psych ward or jail. I read somewhere they hope to eventually have a Zendo outside every psych ward, a lofty goal. They want to divert people from entering the never-ending psychiatric treadmill by giving them a chance to go through the crisis to its end with support instead of focusing on stopping the process. The project has raised hundreds of thousands of dollars to support people who intentionally go into altered states via psychedelics, and unintentionally have a bad trip. People take drugs at festivals to enter into altered states of consciousness and out of their normal mind. Manic people who go into an altered state naturally have to take tranquilizers to stay out of altered states and in normal consciousness. Meanwhile, the war on psychedelic drugs continues. We are not allowed to alter our consciousness unless we are dumbing ourselves down with the likes of alcohol or TV.

The brain makes its own endogenous cannabinoids like anandamide and 2-arachidonoylglycerol.[70] Is the inner pharmacy a mistake in the transcription and translation of the brain's genes? Or do these genes get expressed for a healing process in the psyche? Is mania healing? MAPS, or the Multidisciplinary Association for Psychedelic Studies, has fundraised tons of money, funding studies to test the efficacy of psychedelics like MDMA and psilocybin for PTSD and easing fear of death in studies of those who are terminally ill.[69] Terrance McKenna said, "The way in which these psychoactive compounds that were being brought into the diet were acting, is that they were psycholytic on the formulation of the ego. They literally suppressed the formation of the ego and promoted instead collectivist, tribal, partnership values which were operating intuitionally."[71] Mania is also psycholytic on the formulation of the ego. When the ego is broken up, healing is increasingly possible. Psychedelic states are again becoming more acceptable, and even re-contextualized as therapeutic with controlled clinical and therapeutic protocols. If altered states happen without warning and without a reason, then a brain disease is a likely interpretation, rather than the brain releasing healing inner psychedelics. If exogenous or outside psychedelic substances are now seen as therapeutic and can create healing, maybe endogenous or internal psychedelics made in mania can be healing too.

Imagine we could consciously connect to our ability to affect our inner pharmacy. We can. Think about running. It makes serotonin and generates a runner's high. In the state of mania, our spontaneous, synchronistic actions are making our inner psychedelics. We generate a new symphony of neurochemicals through our perceptions, actions, movements, and gestures. For example, hugging produces oxytocin. Hugging is an action, a gesture. Mania doesn't happen in a vacuum. It happens when we are acting immersed fully in life. We aren't limited to serotonin, acetylcholine, dopamine, epinephrine, norepinephrine, GABA, etc. We produce the endogenous psychedelics plus oxytocin–the bonding neurochemical and hormone. When our endogenous pharmacy makes more oxytocin and endocannabinoids, we see, live in, and create a different world. It's a parallel reality and creation. Think about all the new actions, gestures, and experiences we have and the reality testing we undertake. It creates new neurochemical combinations outside of normal, and we live life outside of normal. We act outside the box of reality and are in a reality outside the box. We can only act our way there to make it happen.

Flow States and Witnessing Overflow

While some people go into an altered state of mania without trying, others try to alter their state of consciousness by all possible means to escape the prison of the mind. A clear illustration of this came in a release from the Flow Genome Project in 2017. They sent an infographic titled "the four trillion dollar a year altered states [of consciousness] economy in the USA."[72] People are spending four trillion dollars on getting into a state that we get into for free and without trying via mania. Without a natural mania, others can only get into altered states that are intense for short periods before it wears off. The body habituates to any outside agent, and the mind undergoes hedonic adaptation to every novel pleasure. We need a bigger and bigger fix. We've been blinded from seeing and experiencing our innate capacity because of our high reliance on outside pleasures.

Mania is a level of consciousness. Some people connect to it and don't need an altered state economy to buy a taste or go on a trip. Manic people rely on the psychiatric economy to tranquilize them from entering mania. Mania is an iterative, chaotic awakening process. Just as psychedelic therapies are being studied to plunge into traumatic experience, go through it, learn from it, and resolve and integrate it, the same can be made true of the non-volitional extraordinary state called mania. During psychedelic therapy, we are encouraged to express what we are experiencing. We have permission to cry unabashedly. The same can't be said for mania when we can't hold it in and out of public view. Our expressiveness is seen as illness. We need more guides and witnesses of the process and less tranquilizers to keep us dulled out. We need people to impartially witness us as we go through our extended process. Sometimes strangers in the community are a witness. They don't judge us, though their perception is being co-opted to see all outcry as an illness.

We need to create a different place for ourselves in consciousness and society. We need to reclaim our mysticism. It's part of our mission to create this. Only we can do justice to what we experienced. And we must do it together because the mission is too big to go it alone. We can do it all-one.

A NEW APPROACH – HARVESTING THE
MEANING IN MANIA

"To invent your own life's meaning is not easy, but it's still allowed, and I think you'll be happier for the trouble."

- Bill Waterson

Engaging Extraordinary Experiences

Traditional biological approaches rely on slow scientific discoveries to create evidence-based treatments in mental health. Recovery-oriented approaches widen to include psychosocial life factors but are limited to practical categories. Our new approach, re-uncovery uses an inner discovery-oriented, psychological, spiritual, philosophical, and informational approach. Re-uncovery asks, what did you discover about yourself and the world from your extraordinary experiences? What new insights do your experiences generate in the moment now? What do you want to move towards and bring into your daily life, not just physically but in your pattern of consciousness? In a way, we are writing over some of our ego programming and deprogramming ourselves from the false-self. Mania rapidly deprogrammed us, and we can use that experience to re-program, code, and re-engineer our consciousness. And as consciousness is the creative factor in life, if we create our consciousness, we create our life.

We no longer ignore our expanded experiences and call them illness to fit into society. Nor is it about trying to fit our expanded experiences back into consensus life. It's about utilizing our extraordinary experiences to decontextualize and recontextualize the meaning of our lives. The clues were planted in our consciousness in mania, and now we can harvest the fruits, participate in our mystery, and solve new puzzles iteratively.

When our power and strength are awakened, we don't put all our worth in recovering what we can salvage from the old way and the old world. We can access and discover the new, anew, now. The new has nothing to do with what we think life is about—which is from thought. 95% of our thoughts are repetitive and repetitive thinking dulls, numbs, and deteriorates the brain.[73] Neuroscience once said we only use 10% of our brain.[74] That was proven to be a myth. It also said that there was no neuroplasticity in the brain after 25. Now they say we use much more of our brain and our brains can grow and change through our whole life. Yet, we had this capacity all along, before science said it. Unfortunately, if 90% of the time we are unconscious, our brain is being used incorrectly. What's the point of using 100% of our brain incorrectly only 10% of the time? We are still in a pickle—like one of those oversized pickles you get at a fair. And maybe we're in this pickle because generations of people thought they couldn't change after 25, so they went on repeating thoughts in their head instead of learning.

What Does it all Mean?

In mania, we have lots of fresh new information arising in our brain mixed in with past thoughts and memories. Our subjective consciousness becomes radically engaged with new information and tries to learn what it means. To try, we naturally have to make creative inferences on the fly. Our approach is meaning alchemized with new information in our subjective consciousness. Whether or not the process is objective or not is not the question. What's essential is the sense of alchemizing new meaning and insights in consciousness through the perceptions of our active, engaged, conscious, and alive brain. Then we see life is full of meaning that we co-create with the present moment. We can only create in the present. We figure into the moment by figuring it out.

What is the meaning of meaning? The definition of the word meaning according to the Merriam-Webster:

PURPORT: the thing one intends to convey especially by language: "Do not mistake my meaning."

IMPORT: the thing that is conveyed especially by language: Many words have more than one meaning.

AIM: something meant or intended: "A mischievous meaning was apparent."

SIGNIFICANT QUALITY: especially IMPLICATION of a hidden or SPECIAL significance: "A glance full meaning."

The logical CONNOTATION of a word or phrase.

The logical DENOTATION or EXTENTION of a word or phrase.[75]

The second definition is "conveying or intending to convey meaning." In mania, life takes on a different significance and intention. Special messages sometimes contain new language elements. They get conveyed as things in time and space. This seems to connote or denote that an influx of meaning is an innate part of the manic state. We start to develop a sense of subjective meaning from perceiving meaning artifacts. We can fine-tune it into a sixth sense. The sense of meaning is subjective and participatory, and this is needed both to sense new meaning and to build our sense of meaning. We learn to walk by walking and making adjustments when we fall. We learn to talk by talking and get feedback from our own gibberish. We learn to sense meaning by sensing meaning and making sense of it in our own way. And then we mean what we say because we've created it. Our words come from the meaning we see now. This is the truthful state. We go on an exploration of building this sense because the planet's ecosystem needs more of us to sense what life means beyond what humans say it means.

Without the participatory sense of meaning, which is also the ability to sense possibilities in the quantum field, we live according to what things meant and what we were told they meant. We search for the meaning of life by going to ashrams, retreats, courses, or by wandering the Earth. The truth is, life is naturally full of meaning, and when our sense of it is first awakened, we feel like we are staring into a bright light. Life is so meaningful and beautiful it's intense and often painful. Imagine if we ran away from the light, back to the darkness because the intensity of the morning sun was too much. If we face it for a moment, we quickly adapt. Maybe we don't adapt as quickly to mania, but perhaps we can if we try. By the way, bipolar people aren't welcome at Vipassana retreats. Some who attend Vipassana retreats land in the psych ward with no prior diagnosis. Although already controversial, it's worth pointing out that you have to sign a long waiver with a detailed section for people with bipolar disorder before attending the Landmark Forum. Some people go manic from the intense workshop. Sean Blackwell wrote a book about his experience called "Bipolar or Waking Up."

Pastures of Meaningful Dialogue

Speaking of bright light, one time, I was having a dialogue with a friend about Krishnamurti's teachings. We were in a spiritual environment. While reading a passage, inquiring deeper, and asking each other questions, suddenly, the whole room changed to look like a golden-green hologram. We looked at each other, and after a few seconds, we both had to avert our eyes. We kept trying to look at each other, but it was too intense, and our heads would turn, like two strong magnets coming together only to be pushed away. We both realized love was present, but our human bodies were not accustomed to the bright light in each other's eyes—the light of love. In life, we turn away from each other because we are afraid of love. Because we are afraid, love is not. Love is intense.

I remember Dr. David Bohm once saying we don't have feelings: we have "felts." Our emotions are a repetition of a feeling we've felt many times. They are habitual. We get triggered into feeling our felts. Using the same logic, we don't experience the meanings of life, but what it "meant." We can't sense the significance or meaning of each moment now because we've already been told what it meant through words and definitions. We think we already know what the moment means but instead of accessing the infinite possibility of what the present moment means, we experience what is meant through repetitive thoughts, associations, images, and memories. We experience our projections on the moment rather than the moment itself.

Control the Inner Chatter in a Box?

Chatter defines our world, and we live in a box of those definitions. We are boxed in by our projections and away from love. We can't contact or see the undefined infinity of eternity. Our world is a chatterbox. What we are meant to experience as life is pre-programmed into us to keep us domesticated with little need to think for ourselves. Life isn't a program. Life is what it means now, afresh, to an uncluttered and attentive brain-body-heart-eye-hand-consciousness. Consciousness is the coordinator. The moment and nature are the conductors. The Universe is well-meaning and to see meaning is wellness.

Scientific experiments show our brain initiates actions before we are consciously aware we intend to perform that action.[76] Oddly enough, this applies to the waking state we call "being in control." Science shows something is controlling us before we are even aware of it. The implications are profound. It means our actions are pre-programmed before we are aware, and we have no control. Our very being is being controlled. We don't own ourselves. We are infected. In mania, to an outside observer, we can seem like we are out of control, but that's because we've never been in control during regular waking consciousness and are now trying to figure out what action really is and what freedom really is. Being free of programming is challenging. Every moment presents a new challenge, and we can't rely on habit to respond to it. Being controlled by programs and habits is much easier. It takes less attention. We can afford to let our mind wander. We are controlled by thoughts of should, must, comparisons, false desires, memories, etc. The pre-programs usurp whatever we'd do naturally. It is natural and normal for us to act unnaturally, while it's unnatural and abnormal to act naturally. We are so unaware of our programming—that controls us and keeps us on a tight leash below our awareness—that touching our natural state and trying to master it, without training wheels is called illness.

The Matrix is 'Real' Meaningful

The main issue is that in mania, we are outnumbered by the people still "in the matrix." "The Matrix Delusion" is a term created to invalidate the experience in mania of seeing the masses sleepwalking through life and getting creeped out by it. I think *The Matrix* was created from the truths of altered states. The movie is to send us a message to wake us up. Ironically, since it's a movie, we think waking up to a bigger truth applies only to entertainment on the silver screen. The film helped people who go into mania and psychosis to put words to what we were already experiencing. By saying 'Mania feels like *The Matrix*' or that we feel like we are in the matrix when we are in mania, we can easily articulate it to others. *The Matrix* is a metaphor, but the film wasn't released before the existence of mania or psychosis. If one has delusions for forty years, then gets labeled with The Matrix delusion after watching it, is that even valid? Since we haven't created our understanding, we hitch onto other understandings and piggyback off metaphors in films so others can understand us. Our attempt to communicate is turned into a delusion. We need to create more language to describe our experiences for ourselves. Many creative works, music, movies, poetry, and more were fueled by creators taking psychedelics or purely by "madness." Their art can help us communicate what mania is like, because it's like being on psychedelics, which is like being mad. Many movies besides *The Matrix* depict certain experiences that can occur in mania, though they are not movies about mania. Again, this is where experiences that have entertainment value are relegated to entertainment while people who experience them are shoved to the psych ward. We all miss out on the gifts while others profit from them and imply that they are only fantasy. It's the same as putting toxic chemicals in food that cause physical diseases, then producing drugs to manage them.

Meaning and Memes

But we were talking about meaning. How do we approach meaning? We create, integrate, and re-contextualize manic experiences to harvest its memes. Memes are bits of culture and meaning transferable through text, voice, and behavior. They are the meaning and cultural equivalent of genes because they are passed on and replicated. Some memes catch on while others don't. The word "selfie" is a meme. The shuffle dance is a meme. Unless we pass on our memes from mania, we will always face oppression from stronger and more replicated memes of the consensus world and psychiatry. Our memes are missing from culture because we've been dismissed. As such, our culture is missing much of what the Universe intended to enculturate us with here in the West. Other world cultures do not ignore this class of memes and have Shamans to make sense of them for everyone. Think of psychiatry as a dominant pool of memes that will always engulf us unless we create a bigger, richer pool of memes. No meme is insignificant because it's needed for the crowding out process. The system is helping us in the ways it knows. It's up to us to figure it out in the ways that only we can know. Building understanding has far-reaching implications. When we create our vast pool of memes and draft bipolar consciousness as something other than just and illness, we will naturally create different roles.

Many of the top-paying jobs today didn't exist ten years ago.[77] The job of being a mental patient has been around for a couple of hundred years now. Our job has created many jobs and fed many families over the centuries—psychiatrists, nurses, psych nurses, pharmacists, pharmacy assistants, pharmaceutical companies, pharmaceutical reps, occupational therapists, organic chemists, clinicians—all those needed to run mental institutions, fill up ice baths, prep lobotomy rooms, icepick manufacturers, and so forth. It's time we start fabricating new roles to play. Maybe it begins like a fantasy roleplaying game we play with each other just for fun to try it out. We can trade our own currency or memes from our experiences. We need to harvest, transcribe, and translate to create the fruits of our experience and find ways to get the profits back in our pockets. It is possible. Can we create the top five jobs for ourselves, besides mental patients?

A Meaningfulness Approach

Another part of our approach is meaningfulness. Meaningfulness is different from mindfulness. Mindfulness attempts to be aware of and pay attention to sensations and feelings in the moment without judging or interpreting them. We are asked to be aware of and pay attention to the content from the past arising in our awareness. If the judge comes in, as it inevitably does, the judge is also the past. When we accept the mind chatter without judging it, we witness meaningless chatter consciously. We may also experience quietness when the chatter subsides for a time, and there is no content to witness. The three possibilities are: unconscious as the judge or past, conscious witness of the unconscious chatter content, or conscious of quietness.

On the other hand, meaningfulness is the next step, where the mind is naturally filled with meaning. We empty the mind of the ego chatter and the ego's sense of life as meaningless so we can be filled with meaning and the sense of meaningfulness. In mania, the mind is full of content that feels fresh and meaningful. Meaning can be an idea, insight, noticing, perception, musing, or wondering. It can be synchronicity. Meaning feels wonderful, exciting, and magical. Meaning is infinite, so we can let go of meaning and trust that more meaning will arise. In mindfulness, we attend to the meaninglessness that our mind is full of in hopes that it will go away. There is a hidden intention of resistance, even if it's supposed to be without judgment, like when our focus is concentrated on a single point to attempt to eliminate everything else. We resist our addiction of attending to the repetitive chatter. While mindfulness tries to resist judgment, meaningfulness activates the subjective alchemy of meaning.

Meaningfulness is an awareness of rich, potential meaning present in each moment, tapping into the source, and playfully participating. Meaningfulness is the opposite of focusing or concentrating on a single point to ignore everything else. Meaningfulness is expanding our awareness equally over the entirety of our senses and field of vision so that which is meant to come into awareness, arises without being blocked by our false will, choice, or concentrating on one point. The ego is always concentrating on one point, itself. It doesn't come close to representing life as it is. We can expand our consciousness and perceptual field to be homologous to the Universe and the Gaian mind. We don't choose what meaning comes. It's not like a train of thought. It's alive. We let the moment 'choose' for us, impress upon us, and we enter the flow of meaning. Universe has more to offer than the ego. It puts the "choice" in the hands of the Universe and wholeness, rather than the separate abstracting self. Then it's not a choice. We enter the flow of life. We trust in everything to bring us something. Our being is the moment, and the moment is meaning. How can something new come to us from everything if we focus on a point of our choosing that looks at the past?

Is this a Meaningful Universe?

How is it possible for the infinite Universe not to bring something meaningful? That's the ego's job. The false-self is the only thing that makes a lack of meaning possible. The false-self is a limiter that limits our meaning and experiences by keeping us one thought away from connecting with actual life instead of its abstractions and projections. Actual life is not after our next thought: it's before the thought you're about to think. Can we abide there? When we are not in touch with our infinite nature, we are blocked because we focus our sacred attention on meaningless thoughts that clog up our awareness. We can only pay attention to what's meaningless or meaningful at any given time. When the ego chooses instead of Gaia, life is meaningless. When we are grounded in awareness, and our attention is relaxed, life comes to play with us. We live in a playful Universe. One helpful practice is to relax your eyes while looking straight ahead, then look around the room out of your peripheral vision without moving your eyes. Look at a point, but don't focus on it, or concentrate. Activate all the 'dots' of your field of vision with your conscious attention. When we spread our awareness evenly over our visual field, the Universe can 'choose' what we see. Our whole visual field is alive. Something will catch our eye, and it'll be a surprise. It's life. We see life first.

In mania, life feels meaningful because it's new. It's a truth that life is always new. We are learning the art of living with the factual sense that life is always new, and therefore meaningful. In short, we are connected with the source. The source is eternally original, and we are that. Now is the time to normalize NEW. The time has come to be original, to be in the newness. In other words, we need to make originality in perception the rule rather than the exception. Mania is a mutation and metamorphosis back to our originality. Mania is originality embodied. It's easy and natural to be original and spontaneous in mania. We have lots of energy when we live from our origin. Being super original is a heroic act—it's micro-heroism.

Originality is our birthright, yet we've been anything but. Consider how much warped and distorted energy there is in the world because we weren't our original selves acting in the majority of moments. Multiply that by 7 billion people. We can see why the world is the way it is. Mania is a course correction heuristic from this cognitive dissonance. The violence needed to suppress and second-guess ourselves accumulates and results in violence in the world. Our original self is needed to remedy the situation. Mania is a solution to the collective distortion; the accumulated relativity and gravity of all our missed moments. There is a real Earth somewhere, and we ain't on it. The Universe is calling us to wake up and be original. Mania answers the call and gives us the energy to be fearless, original, and spontaneous. The solution state is to be original in the present moment. Our being is meaning when we live in the moment.

Surfing the Tsunami of Consciousness

One of the functions of the manic waves of energy is to force us to learn to surf the tsunami of consciousness and overcome our sheeple domestication. We can share our harvests as we glean many of the same themes, thoughts, principles, values, and workings of reality in the process. We understand that this is evidence of a weird quantum world and a brain adapting to it, not an ill brain. We need to create channels to communicate that aren't about symptoms or side effects, but about re-languaging, re-wording, re-contextualizing, re-writing, and re-gaming our collective narrative, life, and culture. There are meaningful special messages, ideas, insights, memes, innovations, perspectives, visions, dreams, synchronicities, possibilities, and impossibilities. We need to have dialogue and step up as "meaning leaders" in our community.

In a video by Andrew Moskowitz called *Is Psychosis Meaningful?* he says, "Against the view of madness as 'incomprehensible' comes the position that psychotic symptoms are not only meaningful but that their meaning must be understood for genuine healing to occur."[78] This goes for mania too. We need to share the meanings we have stored in our notebooks, brains, audio, and video recordings to balance warped energy. Our purpose is meaning, and we can mean well. When we weave enough meaning, there will be an emergent property—an epiphenomenon. A participatory theory of meaning is when we don't rely on the meaning from the dictionary or human constructs but create it in participation with Gaia in the present. When we have a direct relationship with Gaia, we don't need much else. Meaning is your interface and your inner-face. How do we change our orientation to meaning now rather than ruminating?

Over time, we will upgrade our system to the bipolar subjective meaning meta-processing heuristic to process our bipolar experiences after the fact. Manic consciousness needs to create the tools that manic consciousness needs to create the next evolution in manic consciousness. Otherwise, we will always be on the psychiatric "medication maintenance" treadmill, trying to recover into a meaningless cookie-cutter life. Eventually, we won't need to meta-process mania after the fact. We will eternally live with the fact of life—that it's always fresh, new, and original. We'll have designed our brain to live with life. The beauty of the origin is in the eye of the beholder. And with this, you are beholden to the Universe and as the Universe. You are beloved. You are, be loved. Love being human because you are love being human.

WORDS ABOUT WORDS – RE-LANGUAGING BIPOLAR DISORDER ON OUR OWN TERMS AND IN OUR OWN TERMS

"Is it possible for human beings to bring about a totally different category or dimension of the mind?"

- J. Krishnamurti

Re-Languaging 947 Pages of Oversimplified Complications

The DSM categories for bipolar diagnoses are oversimplifications designed for doctors and clinicians. The lived experiences are much more complex. To say that bipolar is up and down or a high or low mood isn't the whole story. It might be useful for us to reconsider the term bipolar altogether. This strategy can double in that it can reduce the self-stigma and stigma. The lived experiences aren't just between two poles, either good or bad. We could better describe it as omni-directional and omni-dimensional. "Omni" means "all." We have access to new rich sensations, experiences, feelings, and emotions. It's as if we have access to all of them and more. I coined the word "omnipolar" to denote including all poles on the spectrum of being human. To me, omnipolarity gives us access to more of what it means to be human, not more of what it means to be ill or less of what it means to be human. We are called ill because we have access to disallowed aspects of human consciousness and experience. There is human potential and experience, known and unknown, in this dimension or parallel realities, and everything in between, infinity and eternity. It's as if the gates to our multifaceted beingness open up. Once we've seen this truth with our own eyes, and been there in our own body, we can't forget or unlearn this.

We can re-contextualize the notion of a persons' 'relapse of illness' to a persons' 'reoccurrence of possibilities.' Depression after mania is grieving the loss of possibilities. The diagnosis process works to catch us at particular points of our experience with a small net of symptoms that gives the trained eye the right to capture and diagnose us for life. The small subset of clinically created symptoms that apply to a tiny fraction of the experience is justification enough to reduce us to an illness and make us into a mental patient forever. If they took any other subset of our experiences and treated us well accordingly, we could be made into something else. As it is, we have to make something else of ourselves for ourselves.

We can do better for ourselves. Re-languaging is important because words have immense power. The way we speak colors how we experience life. How we speak about ourselves is how we experience ourselves and create ourselves. A small language change can create a vastly different trajectory over time. An airplane flying just one degree off course while traveling halfway around the equator will be 250 miles off target.

We've already talked about reclaiming the word "mania" from pathology and placing it in alignment with positivity as it's used in most contexts. Perhaps we need a completely new word to describe the majority of mania that is beyond and has nothing to do with pathology or the small net of capture-criterion. We need a word to connote the actual living experience of it by experiencers. Perhaps "omnia," which looks close to mania, and includes omni, as in omnipolar. Another possibility is "amnia" which is related to amnion. Amnia contains the same letters as mania rearranged. Amniotic is related to a growing embryo, yet to be born. Perhaps we are growing the embryo of our possible self each time we go into mania. Maybe to be psychotic is to be "amniotic."

Another word for mood is "spirits." Another way to say, "I'm in a good mood," is to say "I'm in good spirits." "Mood swings" then becomes "spirit swings." A mood disorder then is a spirit disorder. This sounds much closer to the truth. When we appear moody to others, our spirit is trying to breakthrough. Many of us report having a whole array of spiritual experiences. In English we say, "I am angry." In Spanish they say, "I have anger." We are a spirit, but we are not a mood. I can say I have a spirit, or I am a spirit. Our spirit is made up and inclusive of many moods and modes. The spirit is also beyond mood and emotion. The spirit is omni, or all. I suppose it's easier to justify medicating a mood more so than a spirit.

Neologisms as a Strength

This subtle change in the language has big implications. If there isn't a good word to describe or encapsulate something we experience, we can propose or coin a new one. The word for coining new words is "neologism." Neologisms are one of our strengths. It makes sense because our experiences outside the box defy the limits of our current language inside the box. In the psychiatric framework, neologisms are considered a symptom of bipolar or schizophrenia, not a strength. That's when it's up to our subjective alchemy to re-contextualize. Not only can we re-contextualize, but we can also reclaim some of what's included in the DSM-5 under bipolar as part of the illness and reframe it as a strength according to living experience. Let's take neologisms. Neologisms are in the DSM-5 as a symptom of illness. We can recognize and declare the ability to create words and language as a strength and even a necessity. Re-contextualizing neologisms as a strength is an example of a symptom in the medical context being an important trait in our own context. We don't have to fight the DSM and get them to remove neologisms as a pathological symptom in order for us to use neologisms on our path. We can shift any symptom to a strength and use them as we need. Any symptom can be seen as a strength from a different perspective or from the experience of a different dimension. If you think about the psych ward intake questionnaire, which includes asking about special messages, reading others' thoughts, psychic ability, seeing things that 'aren't there,' and lots of energy, maybe it speaks more of clues to some of the abilities that we can learn to master. The consensus world doesn't want us to know about them or master them because empowered beings can't be oppressed or programmed.

We can also derive new perspectives and lived experience lenses by peering into words that are currently used. Bipolar is far from predominantly being a pathology. At the same time, "pathology" can be re-languaged to "the study of the path," because "ology" means "the study of." Path-ology. Diagnosis can be re-languaged and recontextualized to "dia-gnosis" or "across knowledge of spiritual mysteries." So sometimes we don't need new words, just wordplay, new context, and an inner trust in our truth, our validity. 'Bipolar' is a quality of light and experiencing bipolar is like seeing a world of light versus a world of darkness. The light world is like energy, and the dark world is like matter. If I take myself to be a light being, then bipolar is a nice descriptor.

What is known is known through language. Making new words with new intentionality changes the fabric of subjectivity, salience, and reality. Even if it initiates the placebo effect, the placebo effect is the power of human attention and intention. It's not inert, it's more powerful than the material. It could be, if we designed our linguistic "placebo" we might rid ourselves of the need of medications because in studies, many don't work much better than a placebo. It could be that the disempowering language and education of psychiatry is necessary for the medications to work at all through the belief in them, by bring us down to that vibration. If there was a system to help us vibrate higher because of our experiences, medications would only bring us down. Why do they take so long to "work?" Is it because when we are fully demoralized, we surrender?

The Right to Play with Language

Let's look at an area of human rights where changing language is being encouraged. Look at all the strides made describing gender diversity, considering what individuals are experiencing in their consciousness and being, despite the traditions of consensus reality. Here is a group of people telling the world the exact terms by which they request to be referred to, and people are finally listening. They are creating new words all the time to make distinctions, expand diversity, validation, and aid communication. Some people identify as "gender fluid." Maybe we are "consciousness fluid?" I've even thought of myself as "neuro-fluid." I've mentioned the word "trans-conscious" instead of bipolar because it feels like transitioning between two modes of consciousness. Sometimes I'm in the old paradigm Newtonian ego consciousness, and other times in new paradigm manic quantum consciousness. I can transition between the two. Why can't we have diversity of consciousness that has nothing to do with gender or sexuality, and everything do with the rest of life? I'm sure I can create some pronouns so people can refer to me based on the state of my consciousness rather than what bits I may or may not have or who I want to sleep with. How about "oc" for omnipolar consciousness? Or "bibs" for bipolar Bodhisattva. I don't have to be she.

People diagnosed on the Autism spectrum proclaim they are a neurotribe full of neurodiversity.[79] They want less to be fit into a box and more to be understood as being fine without the box, with unique abilities and ways of processing information. We might call ourselves a trans-conscious or omnipolar neurotribe with unique abilities, ways of processing information and rapid shifts in processing and behavior. We are shapeshifters. We can create our own distinct magic words to paint pictures of our diverse, fluid consciousness for others. As it is, our consciousness is called mentally ill. It's up to us to make new distinctions.

We can re-langauge the negative connotations around 'glorifying mania.' We aren't trying to glorify part of an illness. We are glorifying our actual lived experience of consciousness, energy, information, spacetime, meaning, mystery, magic, eternity, the quantum, the unknown, synchronicity, and being alive as a human. Mania makes the unfolding of life feel significant again. It feels like the end of an eternal quest to find ourselves and the beginning of living life as ourselves. We try to point out and communicate the beauty and meaning that we notice to others. We see a lot and say a lot. Often, others can't see what we see and take our musings and shenanigans the wrong way. They think something is wrong with us because we see, experience, and act differently; especially when we were 'normal' before.

Allies for Expression of Inner Experience

How about joining in the fun? We would love allies, just like LGBTQIA+ people. LGBTQIA+ allies don't necessarily know what it's like to be lesbian, gay, bi, or trans, but they help to empower them knowing they have a right to be who they are. I think we are being who we are told we are—mental patients, and who wants to be referred to as that? We need fewer clinicians and more allies. We can be who we are beyond these oppressive ideas. For this, we must venture into the unknown.

Can we create our own philosophy? Not Eastern or Western Philosophy, but Manic Philosophy? Possible forms of inquiry include 'intra-mania' or looking inward at the manic process. Retro-mania or meta-mania is processing a mania after it's over. Processing the information may lead to ultra-mania or a mania that is integrated and less hyper-mania. These are all proposed neologisms. Eventually, we can share our philosophy with non-experiencers, neurotypicals, and a-manics. "They" are guests, visitors, listeners, and possible allies. Through dialogue, we can unfold meaning and create mutual upliftment to bridge the gap. Can we be CHAMPION Navigators? Rearrange the letters and get MANIC HOP Navigators—navigating hopping between manic and mainstream worlds. Okay, maybe I'm getting a bit carried away. But that's me being a little bit manic all the time.

We need to create words to describe what we do. An overarching term for our work to bring manic magic to the masses could be

"Manicians" or "Alchemanicians." The more manicians we have, the less clinicians we'll need. We can be steppingstones for each other. Let's, as manicians, make sense of our information and discuss it amongst ourselves. We may find a way to make our mission a reality. Manic Trans-Consciousness has something to say to everyone. If we can put aside the experiencism, languagism, and perceptionism biases towards bipolar mania and psychosis, we can share a glimpse. We can be as we are and do what we came here to do.

SELF-DIALOGUE FOR RE-UNCOVERY

"I already spoke this into existence."

- Ralph Smart

Creating Meaning through Dialogue in Consciousness

In 2016, I started having a dialogue with myself. That dialogue was key to unlocking the meaning in mania. What I call Self-dialogue is a safe container to look at the information, meaning and experience of mania. Through dialogue, you can harvest your mania, create consciously, and live your dreams. Dialogue is all about communicating to unfold meaning.

Dr. David Bohm said, "The point is that dialogue...goes into the process of thought behind the assumptions, not just the assumptions themselves."[80] He also made another important distinction in dialogue when he said, "Dialogue may not be concerned directly with truth—it may arrive at truth, but it is concerned with meaning."[80] That's why Self-dialogue is so powerful, because it gets behind the assumptions of thought and gets into meaning. The mental health system gives us a quick "truth" that we are mentally ill to explain our experiences. Dialogue is concerned with our meanings, not some arbitrary, "objective" truth. Luckily, we can use dialogue as a powerful tool for ourselves.

In a way, mania itself is a dialogical state of consciousness because we can shift between many points of view and perspectives and discover new meaning. Sometimes we talk just to talk to ourselves or have dialogue with what we see, whether it's a tree, person, or a fly. Other people can think we don't consider others when we are in dialogue with many things at the same time. Life isn't just about people. They can think we don't make sense, but what we are saying has subjective meaning to us. Everything feels meaningful because we can't discern what is 'more or less important,' and that's precisely why we can see meaning everywhere. We don't filter based on our past programming. We talk a lot because we are in a dialogue of meaning.

Dr. David Bohm wisely said, "A change of meaning is a change of being."[81] Through dialogue, creating meaning is essentially creating our being. But who are we going to have dialogue with? I remember reading in Bohm's book, *On Dialogue*, that if there is no one to have a dialogue with, have a dialogue with yourself. I read that after I'd been having a dialogue with myself for one and a half years. I knew I was on the right track. Re-uncovery or meta-mania is engaging our manic ideas, insights, and experiences through Self-dialogue. Self-dialogue is exactly as it sounds— we have dialogue with ourselves. In mania, we are in a Self-dialogue. We are communicating with many things. Our usual communication with the people we know goes down the tube, but we can talk with anything else, even grass. Self-dialogue isn't about our internal chatter or trying to think better thoughts. The chatter of the ego is full of discussion, debate, and conflict. We aren't trying to make the ego process, which relies on debate and conflict, better. The ego can't do dialogue, though we can dialogue with the dead elements of the ego. The ego isn't alive because life is not repetition.

Relax Your Attention by Speaking in a New "Tense"

We will engage a new mode of speaking with ourselves, our manic content, and the Universe. Self-dialogue is like a new tense of language. It's a way to go into the past, present, and future in the content of consciousness in the present. I've developed a process to understand my extraordinary experiences that doesn't rely on anyone else. I'm sharing my understanding with you so you can use any building blocks that you like. The power lies in building your interpretations, meaning, and context. By engaging in dialogue, and putting our consciousness in a dialogical state, we are being a little bit manic and going beyond the illness paradigm that says don't bother. That's the only step. If we see this is our real consciousness, we can solve any problem because we are communicating with the source from the source. We are already orienting our attention in our capacities.

I started talking to myself and the Universe on a consistent basis in June of 2016, and I continued for three years. I documented 700 hours of dialogue on video. That 700 hours amounted to 1.7 million words. That's enough words for 42 books. Had I attended talk therapy I'd have a $70,000-$140,000 bill. Self-dialogue is free, for you, by you, when you want. It's a powerful tool to talk yourself into the being the 'you' who you know you are, especially if you had mania. While most therapy tries to get us to fit into the world, Self-dialogue builds our map and territory of consciousness that can be the ground that we stand on, the mountain we climb up, and the ground we come crashing back down on. You will discover and be empowered by your own inner and outer voice. You will see directly that the process of life will reverse for you, from outside in, to inside out, because of dialogue. When you have a dialogical mind, that's the way life works because you are in a relationship with life. It communicates with you not just through words but through experience, just like it does in mania. First, we discover something, say it, then the Universe can show us we are on the right track through feedback and feedforward. It indeed works in mysterious ways, and you are part of the mystery. We will see the Universe is communicating with us because the odds of many successive synchronicities are small. When something comes to our awareness, then that exact thing happens in our experience within a day or so, it's just too obvious. It seems like life is designed to be designed for us, and it is. When we've seen it with our own eyes it's insane to continue to think we don't have direct, participatory communication with the Universe. We'll have too much evidence from what the Universe makes evident. You'd think it'd be more subtle, and it is the subtle that is for us.

Logorrhea to Logos

The first time I was manic, I experienced it as an extraordinarily profound and magical time filled with mystery and synchronicity.

I made some recordings of me talking, and who knows how much of it made sense or would make sense if I listened now. Even if it didn't make sense, it didn't matter because I was testing what was coming to mind by speaking it out loud, much like a child sounds out words to learn to read. As the child makes the first sound, the second, then the third, they then know what word they are reading. If they don't sound out the word, they may never read the word or the sentence. In mania, we sound out a different source of words, sentences, and meanings from the Universe. And we don't really need to know what we're going to say. The same process by which a child learns a language, bipolar people create new language. We do this by talking without ego-filtering or thinking first, sounding out the Universe, and being okay or perhaps oblivious to the awkwardness and vulnerability of our speech. At the same time, this is a type of reality testing of language, and we are talking to the Universe. The Universe doesn't judge language like humans do. The Universe gets excited when humans start sounding out never before uttered chaos into emergent language. Additionally, this builds the brain's neural networks so we can commune with the new source. We can lay the foundation so that others can connect to the source too. The trouble is that others notice our awkwardness and think something is wrong with us. For now, it's better to practice writing and speaking as we do in private. It's important to integrate the information and meaning overload.

During my first mania, I wrote out 700 pages by hand. Much felt like channeling or automatic ('automanic') writing. It continued for two months, then I was hospitalized. The psychiatrist told me I had bipolar disorder with psychotic features, a meaningless brain chemical imbalance. You may recall that my first thought was "that's not it." I knew it wasn't the time or place to argue, but that state of meaning has stayed with me since. I didn't start taking an alternative look at things until three years later. That's when I found books that showed I wasn't alone in my perspectives. My first mania wasn't the only time I'd receive a huge download of information. I went on to experience mania a handful more times. What was I to do with all the persistent information? Self-dialogue was my way to process the information overload. Since then, I've been learning and creating meaning daily and I'd like to share what I've discovered with you. Sensing and making meaning is a skillset. We will hone our meaning making abilities to extrapolate meaning from almost anything at a glance.

Dialogue to Trialogue

Self-dialogue is more like a trialogue. The trialogue is between our being, the Gaian mind or Universe and manic meanings and perceptions. We run our thoughts, ideas, insights, and experiences by the Universe with our own voice and look out for relevant feedback and feedforward. If we don't give voice to our insights, we can't get validation and creation from Gaia. The human voice is the most powerful instrument in the Universe. It's creative. First, there was the word, right? We need to get our words right. Researcher Don Estes found that the voice says more about us then we know:

> We've done years of researching human biometrics (brainwave/ neuromapping/heart rate variability monitors) but we've discovered you can understand more about who a person is and what they want from their voice than from their brain or

their heart. The brain shows how they're thinking about it and the heart shows how they're feeling about it but the voice shows immediately all those things. You can hardly change your state of mind without it showing up in your voice. And if you think about it, it makes a lot of sense because the voice is the mechanism the Universe gave us to say who we are and what we want.[4]

Elsewhere, Don Estes points out the difference between the instrument and the player, where the exact same saxophone can be played by two different players, and the feeling behind it is much different.[4] We manics are working on our voice instrument, the feeling of it resonating through our body, and creating the true player of our body-voice-instrument. We need to build our own voice because the false-self has been using our instrument. Our so-called normal inner voice is a combination of the voices of many people, disguised as our thoughts, because it's recorded and transformed by the brain into the sound of our voice in our head. If people start to hear intrusive voices, they are usually the sound of someone else's voice. We don't realize the sound that we think with, the one we believe to be our own voice, is an intruder too. The experience of another's voice speaking our thoughts as happens in schizophrenia could be closer to the truth than our regular experience where we hear our thoughts spoken in the sound of our own voice. When we hear them as our own voice, we don't realize they are intruders, or parasitic memes, even though they come from the voice of another person in our formative years. Going through the process of ceasing to believe what thoughts say, whether as our voice or as another's, can bring some relief.

Voices of Difference and the Dialogical
Voice of Equals

People's voices have infected us when we record something they say. We get a life sentence of other people's sentences. "You're not good enough," blah, blah, blah. We've received information from the outside and assimilated and recorded in the sound of our own voice. We call this normal though our whole consciousness is occupied by thought viruses from others. It uses our own machinery, our own voice, to perpetuate itself, just like viruses use the hosts DNA to replicate itself. Are we hearing voices because we are being used by voices heard as other or disguised as our own? The memes replicate and repeat themselves by using our organism. We aren't using our voice, period. We are being used. We aren't the player. We are being played. I'm going to show you how to change this. You will trust in yourself again and be the author of your own life.

Our new dialogical voice takes a bit of time to learn. Dialogue exercises our voice to connect us with our original voice–our voice when we speak from the origin–until the two become one. This is the gap that we are closing–it's in consciousness. We begin to speak from, with, and as the moment or source. Then our voice is original. Speaking as the moment is like thunder and lightning. First, we see a flash of light or insight on our mindscreen, and then there is a slight delay before our mouth and voice start sounding out the words in material reality. Words cease to arise from choosing from the train of thought. We can also learn to discern who to share our voice with and who not to. We don't have to share our insights with everyone. When we deeply engage with our rich process of

Self-dialogue or meta-mania, we don't feel the urge to say it to everyone or anyone because we've talked it out with the Universe.

Dialogue is meant to be a conversation among equals. To dialogue with the Universe is to be equal to it. We need to be equal to the Universe to hear it. When we humor chattering thoughts, we aren't on an equal plane with the Universe. And the joke is on us. The Universe has no relationship to chattering thoughts which are abstractions. Look at the Universe and see that it's true. Mania levels the playing field. We are used to approaching life as separate and divided from the Universe, which is a false approach. A false approach to the Universe creates a false, illusory reality—one where we are divided from it. Only our perception needs shifting because what's true has always been true. When we speak as the ego and of its chatter, we can only get an illusory reaction from the illusory reality. The ego talks to itself. The me talks, and the self listens. My-self. But who is the "me" and who is the "self?"Are there two of us, or is this another catch-22 that we are stuck in? Think about it. When we speak with Gaia, we have access to the Gaian mind, because there is a response from Gaia. Now, energy is not wasted in illusion, so there is lots of energy to show us more than we've ever imagined in the Universe. It matters who you are speaking as and who you are speaking to. We can speak as one, as the moment to Gaia, not as a false ego to a false-self.

The Practical Potential of Gaialogue

Dialogue is an approach to unfolding meaning. Meaning is a subtle form of matter and entangles with matter. When we integrate meaning, we have access to a wider array of possibilities. When we question assumptions, we open up to the unknown. When we can look from many perspectives, we see the world through many lenses. Through us, the world and Gaia see themselves. We become the eyes of Gaia through the alchemy of human attention. Not only are we using the transformative power of our voice, but the power of our vision too. We are giving voice to that which may have never been said before, if it's not part of the network of repetitive thoughts. When you express your experiences to your doctor, they affirm your diagnosis. When we express to Gaia, we move across knowledge of spiritual mysteries or dia-gnosis. Gaia doesn't pigeonhole you with a label, but she decorates you with meaning. You will find, what you express comes to meet you in manifestation. Life comes to meet you because you are the voice of life itself. Life calls to itself. Life doesn't respond to the ego. Life evolved to speak life into life. Then you are a steward of the voice of Gaia, and you are her friend. You go beyond Self-dialogue and engage in what I call Gaialogue. Recall some of your encounters with nature. If you've contacted nature with your nature, you are nature too. You are a nature mystic when you can speak as nature because nature has a voice of her own that humans can speak.

So here is the process I used to explore manic consciousness with Self-dialogue. Remember, Self-dialogue kept me out of the hospital for three years even though I experienced three major crisis events. The previous three years, I had been in the hospital three times. Six months after stopping the process of Self-dialogue, I ended up in the hospital again. Going into the content of manic consciousness daily prevented a big bang burst of manic energy. We need to saturate ourselves with meaning that we speak with our voice. So how did I do it, and what did I do?

CREATING A MESH OF MEANING IN OUR EXPERIENCES

*"Love will go away if we can't communicate
and share meaning."*

- David Bohm

Cracking the Nutshell with Dialogue

When I was fully engaged in Self-dialogue, a few times a week, I would talk to myself and record it on video whenever I had time. Every day, I wrote down insights as they arose in my consciousness, and then when I had time, I talked them out with myself on video. When I was making the video, I had no idea what I'd end up saying, so when I listened to myself after, it felt like the first-time hearing what I'd said. After recording the video on my iPhone 6s Plus, I used iMovie on my iPhone to edit out the gaps. Listening to what I said while editing gave me more insights and that I would write down. Then, I would talk about those insights in a later video and repeat the process.I published it to a podcast even though it's a rough and raw form, in case documenting the process might help others.

While saying the written insights out loud during the recording process, I would spontaneously expand upon the insights that I had written down and add in more insights. This created a lot of content, and more importantly, context and meaning. I called this process the Triple Extrapolation Process because we can expand on new insights three times to create more insights. Here's how it works:

Step 1   Write down insights during the day as they arise,

Step 2   When there's time, make a video to record yourself talking about the insights. Don't hold back: speak spontaneously without knowing what you're going to say,

Step 3   Listen to yourself talk on the recording while editing out the pauses and write down the new insights you have as you listen to them,

Step 4   Repeat.

During the day, mark down any insights or anything else that has meaning to you in a notebook or electronic notepad. Write it out like raw data. Just this one step validates the fact that new information is trying to alchemize through you into the material realm. You are recording and documenting them, and that's the least you can do. Come back to it later and extrapolate it. Start saying the insight out loud and maybe there's more to it. By recording yourself on audio or video, you capture new insights from your exploring your written insights. Then edit and listen again for more insights, but this time, write them down. It can be done with audio only, though seeing yourself while speaking the insights helps the process. Think about the difference between listening to sports commentary on the radio and watching the game on TV.

You Are Free to Be Your Own Compassionate Witness

There is something to be said about having a compassionate witness to support people through extraordinary states and experiences, just like the Zendo Project does. Since we don't have a witness to support us with our experiences, and if we did it would be too costly, this process is a way we can be a witness for ourselves. It's very powerful. Technology can be an unlimited impartial witness, and we can witness ourselves in the recording. Our phone isn't going to judge us, yet.

Don Estes, who I mentioned earlier, also confirmed the exact process that I discovered for myself as Self-dialogue as evident in this excerpt:

> …because by synchronizing the senses with simultaneous personal harmonic resonance, the information is shared with multiple parts of the brain. For example, if someone says his or her name to you it stores in one place in your brain. If you say it back, it re-distributes to two. If you write it down it is goes to three, and if you look at what you wrote, it gets shared with a fourth. In other words, the more places related information is stored in the brain, the more integrated and useful the information becomes, and the easier it is to recall and utilize as resource. [82]

In the same way, when we do all the steps in self dialogue—writing, speaking, listening, looking—the information is more integrated and useful. And we are drafting and crafting this information ourselves. We are literally filling in the gaps with our voice, eyes, hand, ears, heart, being, and brain. It's the difference between watching someone lift weights and lifting weights ourselves. We are exercising our brain in the direction it's stretching us when we go into mania. We are training ourselves up. The information innervates our being, body, and brain. It's important to build your context to immunize yourself psychologically against any lack of understanding and parasitic memes—information that can live in our brain that is detrimental. Anything you wouldn't think of yourself or identify with by your own choosing is a parasitic meme. Immunize yourself with your own memes, and when more of us do this, we will create 'heard' immunity—immunity to memes we've heard about ourselves but didn't create ourselves through direct perception. Parasitic memes fog up the lenses and perspectives through which we approach life.

While we need to create our own meaning and memes, at the same time, it's important to hold them lightly and not take a strong position on them. This is twofold. One, so we don't start creating a repetitive story that we identify with. And two, so we don't judge or evaluate the memes to keep a steady flow of new memes. In order make meaning and hold it lightly, we can bring in the word "could" as in "it could mean" instead of "it means," which is a way of avoiding being over-certain. 'Could' and 'maybe' assume we don't really know. If we don't really know, then all meanings are held lightly and are thus playful and even fun. In this way, we work to create a sustainable connection to the flow of meaning. Otherwise, we create a small bit of meanings we identify, and this creates a myopathy. Since noise is inversely related to meaning, the more meaning we create, the more the volume of the noise will go down. We usually just try to make all kinds of effort to turn the volume down, but that just adds to the noise through judgement, resistance, and nonacceptance.

The Why's of the Wise

Why use this process:

- Only goal is to create good dialogue and connection with yourself and Gaia
- It's based on free speech and it's free
- To discover the magic of manic memes
- Learn from your own voice
- Upgrading the brain through dialogue
- Learn by speaking as the moment in the moment to the moment
- Perception-action-voice-Gaia is the most powerful feedback/forward system
- Towards more reliance and trust in Gaia
- Build your semantic network based on your experiences
- Self-monitoring augmented by your own understanding
- A way to process information overload
- Increased quality of life
- Accessing neurofluidity
- Less fear of the hospital, and avoid it on some occasions
- A way to integrate, differentiate, and link information
- The Universe will answer without you needing to ask
- Creatively changing cognitive biases and beliefs
- Taking chances in language and language vulnerability

Self-dialogue is a super helpful process for me, and anyone can do it. We need to do this brain-consciousness-Gaia workout several times a week by having Self-dialogue with ourselves. We plan our physical workouts; we need to give our brain cells a metaphysical meta-mania workout. When I saturated myself with my own meaning, I talked myself into my dreams by creating a buffer with my voice between myself and the memes of psychiatry. I had to create a vast mountain of context to overcome the gravity of hundreds of years of psychiatric memes pulling me towards the hospital.

Seeing Through Fear

By talking with myself several times a week about how I saw things, the insights I had, the way I interpreted mental health news, what I was learning about the brain, and more, I created a bubble of meaning and context that crowded out and protected me from identifying with the memes of mental illness. If I started to have "symptoms," my mind would be able to go to places within my voice created context to neutralize the intrusion—like having a memetic immune system. For example, if suddenly my heart started racing, before I might feel like I'm having a panic attack. The fear in my body would increase, and that would increase the likelihood of the panic attack. Then I'd need to take a pill or call for help if it got worse. Without my context and meaning, I'd be hooked into the vicious circle of believing I'm a helpless mental patient. Then I would have a panic attack or full-blown psychosis. Instead, I defaulted to the context I created through Self-dialogue. Talking to myself decreased the fear since I'd fully unfolded so many subtle nuances and possibilities with myself. I was able to outlearn the fear, instead of trying to outrun it. Instead of having a few bits of secondhand clinical knowledge leading me to take fear-based interventions, I had such a vast contextual web so that whatever was happening fit somewhere in it. It fit somewhere into myself, and it wasn't alien to me. I had already taken the time to learn about it. Neutralizing the fear bought me time to create more understanding. I had more time by having a quick dialogue with whatever was happening. The fear was like a pebble compared to my ocean of meaning.

How Not to Write a Book with Your Insights

In addition to the millions of words I spoke with myself to build a mountain of context, I wrote another 700 pages out by hand to seed this book. Not everything I said or wrote out that felt meaningful at the time was also significant. I typed up the ones that still felt meaningful and sorted them into sections. I copied and pasted the significant points into a new document through 11 iterations. I further sorted them into coherent and connected sentences. I don't think anyone recommends writing a book in this way, but it works for bipolar insights. Plus, insights in mania arise in non-linear bits and chunks. I wrote so much in the 700 pages, but none of it was in any order. That's what I had to do manually. It's taken years of building meaning to get to where I am now—trying to pass on a small portion that may be significant to you in this book. More of us need to write books and share our insights. Try sorting yours into sections and putting them in order. Perhaps your special messages add up to a book. Write your own book inspired by this one. Go from noise, to signal, to meaning, and finally significance. What signals or insights arise in your consciousness when you read this book? Do you get a different idea, or does your mind go in a different direction than the one that I go into in the next sentences? Write that down, then triple extrapolate it with Self-dialogue. Write a book. If you think no one will read your book, Google and artificial intelligence (AI) will, and your book will slightly change the internet. Then your memes are on the internet and you've validated what has come to you and through you. If more of us write our books, it will change the internet, even if it's just in a small way. The internet has little representation of our true bipolar world. The psychiatric system prevents us from sharing authentically and programs us to propagate their memes instead of ours.

Triple Extrapolation for Integration

The Triple Extrapolation Process is a way to learn in a self-sufficient way, like an endless fountain that refreshes itself and feels fulfilling within itself. Learning is automatically and intrinsically motivating. We learn for the sake of learning. You can be 95% self-sufficient in creating content, context, and meaning. This decentralizes the source of information that you draw from. We decentralize our consciousness from the very limited network or pool of allowed thought. We become individuals. Beyond self-esteem and self-compassion is self-surprise. The need to endlessly consume secondhand information is minimized. Sometimes when I read information from other people, it generates ten times more insights. If I look at my insights, a bunch more insights are generated. It can lead to information overload to read what others say. At the same time, I can see how their insights relate to my own framework of information.

Through Triple Extrapolation, the newly activated system of energy and information flow in the organism leads to an epiphenomenon—an emergent property or ability that I call

Gaiaence. Gaiaence is Gaia plus Science, where the suffix 'ence' means 'action or process.' Through the education system, we are taught that learning is extrinsic learning. Mania is just one process by which our dormant intrinsic learning abilities re-engage with life. Instead of ripping apart the manifestations of Gaia to find truths, we partner with Gaia in our perceptions as we go about life. The information from our perceptions of the vast possibilities of a Gaia-informed life are intimated inside, intrinsically. Gaia whispers to us and we learn. Triple Extrapolation Process is a part of the Gaiaentific process. Gaiaence is a self-scientific process of intrinsic learning. We can look at life scientifically, with wonder, curiosity, and questions and we will get information to work with. Studies show intrinsic learning is a skill related to empathy, openness to experience, and processing speed.[k] It requires a certain quality of awareness and attention which arises from energy. Then you can understand truths that could be discovered through the scientific method in a glance through wholistic perception. This is partly what's starting to happen in mania, and why we can look at almost anything and it tells us something or gives us a special message. It's communion with what is. You'll have no objective proof, but poof, it's subjectively self-evident. This is a communication. This I call Gaialogue. We are communicating with the moment. It's like our consciousness is gamified. It's a real-life video game. Whatever you look at will tell you what you want to know, or it would like you to know. All of us can do this but we've been made ignorant of our ability to participate with nature and reality. If an emaciated dog came up to us, we wouldn't have use science to understand that it's hungry. Gaiaence is a more subtle version of our ability to know things. In subsequent books we'll build more bridges through understanding implicit learning, big five personality traits, and how apophenia is related to openness to experience, joyous exploration as a big factor in self-actualization, and psychological plasticity.

Philosophy of Gaiaence - Making Hypotheses through Wonder

When I was speaking with myself for three years, I said many surprising things, and some were scientific-ish sounding. I was making hypotheses, theories, ideas, innovations, asking questions—but I didn't look much of it up to see if there was any science to corroborate the stream of words. Learning through perception, downloading, and channeling was too fast. There was just too much to check into it, and my intention was to keep the stream going, not to cut it off by second-guessing Gaia. Recently, I have looked up some hypotheses in scientific journals and it turns out there are already scientific findings related to many of the things I said with Gaia. It shows I'm on the right track. Science made a discovery through the scientific method, and I had an insight to the same discovery, without knowing about the science. The scientific method isn't the only way to make something true, and it doesn't own the truth. I happen to have a Bachelor of Science in Cell and Molecular Biology, so I can read the science. A Gaiaentific mind has more wholistic information because we look at life with Gaia in mind. It's holistic. Gaia doesn't give information so that we can gain power or use it to abuse others. Gaia will tell us if she trusts us. In mania, she's trying to see if she can trust us so we feel like we're being tested. She can't communicate anything to those who want to rip her apart to control her for their profit with the scientific method.

Gaialogue is practical in the above ways and more. I was certain that speaking out loud through Gaialogue had a big impact on my daily life. I kept speaking for 700 hours for the sake of speaking and learning from myself. All of this writing and talking on video has profound practical effects. Don Estes said, "Become aware of how you're being aware. You find out that everything you say comes true. Be careful what you say because those will come back to manifest themselves. That's the bottom line."[82]

We can also look at what we say and watch ourselves speak. I was happy to learn that his research confirmed the Self-dialogue process and writing process I'd been partaking in all those years. It was a consilient finding. Remember, you are talking with yourself, with Gaia, and with the Universe. With life. Everything is alive, is conscious. Gaia will speak to you and through you if you engage with her as an equal. Life is as curious about us as we are about life. Human beings are one of the ways the Universe can be curious about itself. You will see evidence in your life of the power of your voice. Act with your pen and paper. Act with your voice in Self-dialogue. Gaia will bring you synchronicity.

We need to share what we understand about the brain, reality, and life from our own direct lived experience, and we can sort it out through Gaialogue. I talk with my brain and my brain cells. I talk about my brain cells to my brain and with my brain. Turns out, brain cells feed on attention too. How much money is spent on advertising to capture our attention? That by which we are able to pay attention, our brain cells thrive when we give them attention. Our brain cells don't even have our own attention. Our brain isn't imbued with our attention. We are wandering all over the place. Plants grow better with loving human attention in addition to water, soil, and sunlight. If you give your brain cells your attention, they will talk to you and tell you how to release them from the prison cells of thought. If we bathe our brain cells in our attention, they'll grow better. If we put our attention on that by which we are able to attend, we create and access a higher level of consciousness, beyond the brain cells operating in reaction. If we put our attention on the beauty of Gaia, our brain becomes beautiful. Imagine attending to the needs of your brain cells, the actual real cells, instead of your programming. We've been programmed to put our attention on the programming.

Communion with the Gaian Mind

The point here is that we can deduce or extrapolate so much from direct silent observation of the moment, and the moment will tell us what we need to know. We become a channel of higher intelligence. Right now, we don't know that we want to know anything from Gaia. The false-self thinks, therefore it thinks it has better ideas. Communication from Gaia can take many forms. It could be a direct verbal download to the brain that we immediately speak out loud without any forethought, like in transient hypofrontality—or temporary prefrontal cortex deregulation.[83] Transient hypofrontality, where the prefrontal cortex activity lowers and other brain areas predominate may be a common feature in all altered states of consciousness. It may show up in the next email we check, or a random stranger starts talking about it, we see it on a billboard, or it can be a flash of insight that takes weeks to fully unravel in space-time. It can be anything in the Universe's wildest dreams because of your relationship with it. Seeking and searching turn into synchronicity. What a game! Science is too slow for the quantum Gaiaentific brain and eyes. We can know things and others can only wonder how we know or call us crazy instead of listening. When we share what's impossible to know and experience according to the Newtonian framework, we get medicated back to the Newtonian world.

How are the words from Gaia different from words the ego? The higher energy of mania gets rid of any trace of the "silent stutter," a term I heard in the book *The Possibility Principle*. This is where we stutter inside, preforming words out of fear of looking stupid. The book says:

> *Many people feel tentative, if not outright insecure, about sharing their thoughts and feelings. Sensitivity to others' opinions—a symptom of a fragile sense of self and indoctrination in other-esteem—leads such individuals to hesitate. They may vacillate, debating whether to speak, and then question what to share if indeed they choose to make themselves heard. This insecurity interrupts our natural process of articulation, and many people tease out entire sentences in the safety of their own minds before they begin to speak, breaking any sense of spontaneous flow. I think of this halting approach as the equivalent of a silent stutter. Such individuals remain rooted to the principle of certainty.* [53]

Spontaneous Vulnerable Speech – Speaking AS the Moment

Can we master articulation without pre-formation? Sometimes via bipolar, we speak so much that we don't have time to pre-form the words ourselves. It's a sign something else is speaking through us. When we speak preformed and rehearsed words, we are teasing ourselves. We hear words inside of our head before we speak the words out loud. This can lead to the delusion of trying to predict what will happen. Since we hear words inside our heads first, we predict what we say before we say it. The mechanism by which we speak as the false-self—pre-formation—makes us comfortable because we can predict what we will say. This seems simple enough. We preform the words we say, and when we do so, we speak as the past. When we speak the past, we live in the past. We've already preformed the words, and when we did that, the words are coming out from the past, and not the living present. We speak in a predictable way, to ourselves and to others, and that makes us feel comfortable. But we are out of sync with life. By preforming our words, we predict our words, and there is no surprise when we speak.

We like to predict. It's part of what's called Theory of Mind, where we can attribute mental states to others.[84] We can assume why others do what they do. Theory of Mind doesn't work well with someone who is in mania. Sometimes we are seen as selfish and inconsiderate because we aren't playing that game. We are in a different order of operation. To be in the order of the moment, we must speak without preforming. Not only that, while preforming, we can't truly be listening to the moment or another person talking. We can't listen to our own chatter and pre-formation and what others are saying at the same time. Unless we are silent, we can't listen. And unless we listen from silence, we can't speak from silence without pre-formation. It's the ultimate challenge to surrender to silence and not knowing—not even knowing what we are going to say. We are in a Theory of Mind game when we could be in the game of the living present.

When we speak and act without pre-forming, our performance is original, even to us. We must stay in a space of listening, until we hear ourselves speaking words out of our own mouth and are surprised by what we say and do, because it wasn't preformed. Speaking by preformation feeds and sustains the ego games.

This is important because insight comes from a space of uncertainty. Insight is a flash of light that happens in uncertainty. What comes from uncertainty, is certainly truth—from beyond consciousness as we know it. We are attached to certainty, even if it's informationless, energy-less, repetition. We live in, look from, speak from, and react from a mess of projected pre-collapsed wavefunctions. We live in that pre-collapsed state. We aren't open to the now. Here, we are learning to speak from a place of uncertainty. By speaking freely and spontaneously from uncertainty, we are at the same time experiencing our own uncertain words, ideas, and assertions. Speaking from uncertainty should naturally prevent identifying with or being attaching to words. The ego is certain and can come in to make a story out of it. In Gaialogue, we get to the source before and beyond pre-formation. Don't think before you speak. Don't speak as your thinking ego. Don't think, therefore you are not (the ego). Speak as the present moment. Then your voice is a gift to this world.

Tuning in to Share the Universe

And in that way, the Universe is fine-tuning you as an instrument of its communication. To be offensive or on the offense, or be defensive or on defense, both disengage the Universe. We can't be on offense or defense and be curious, in awe and wonder at the same time. To be dialogical is key as we are playing in the field of meaning. We get meaning and significance in our awareness through Gaia and our attention. When we create our own meaning from our perceptions, the Universe knows we got the message.

I hope that one day there will be inclusivity of bipolar experiences and its meaningful interpretations. Dr. David Bohm posed an amazing question when he asked, "Suppose we were able to share meanings freely…Would this not constitute a real revolution in culture?"[85] Freely sharing meanings is not part of our culture, but it is part of the manic culture. We've yet to get to the point where we engage this part of our culture on a larger scale. It's important to pass on meaning through dialogue. When we build shared context, our discoveries help others so that they don't have to suffer and feel informationally alone. We are called ill for what we've discovered. When we re-contextualize our past manic experiences, we also can change the future for all of us because we are editing the consciousness of it. Our meanings are an untapped resource. Making meaning in the present heals. Original meaning entering the brain justifies the existence and purpose of the brain, and it fills the brain with purpose. Learning! We become a constellation of meaning that we have created through a feedback and feedforward loop with the Universe that we can bank on. The brain is a chrysalis for metamorphosis. The ego uses the brain as a ruminant for regurgitation.

Society is not designed for manic consciousness. It's designed for us to be automatons. Just look at the way we are educated. As we walk in mania, we are slowly sinking in the quicksand back to society. Most often, we sink to the lowly place of becoming a mental patient. It's only a disguise for now. One day we will be able to dis-guise ourselves and take off the guise. A guise is an external form, appearance, or manner of presentation, typically concealing the true nature of something. In mania, we live closer to our true nature for a time. Most people never get a chance to touch their true nature at all.

By now, I hope we can see the value of meta-processing our experiences, meanings, memes, and insights with Self-dialogue. When we engage with each other, many more insights will be brought about that could not have been pointed to alone. To really integrate and get to a place where we can make manic consciousness a reality, we must understand the workings of the ego—the false-self. Then it's easier to understand why mania feels more real than life before mania.

Chapter 4

TWO STEPS BACK TO EGO CONSCIOUSNESS

OUR UNNATURAL NATURAL STATE - UNMASKING THE FALSE-SELF AND THOUGHT

"…the ego begins to take hold at first as a kind of cancerous aberration but then quickly becomes a new style of behavior which quickly then eliminates all other styles of behavior by suppressing access to the chaos. This is the point I want to make. That there is between the ego and full understanding of reality a barrier, a problem, the fear of the ego to surrender to the fact of chaos. Chaos is what we have lost touch with…because it is feared between the dominant archetype of our world which is the ego which clenches because its existence is defined in terms of control."

- Terence McKenna

Room and Bored in a World of Mediocrity

It's time to intentionally derail the manic momentum we've built. Like the inevitable expected surprise of psychosis, we are throwing ourselves for a loop. And like a rollercoaster with an upside-down loop, what's the point if we can't enjoy the ride. We're going to explore the ego in the context of bipolar. There are many books that explore the ego or false-self, so we don't need to be exhaustive here. We are going to consider the ego's structure in contrast to the manic state as well. One poignant example is Ryan Holiday's book called *Ego is the Enemy*. We don't get a lesson on the ego in grade school or in the psych ward. I'm not a psychologist or expert but jesting on the gist of the ego is an entertaining endeavor. Learning about the ego after mania is categorically lame in comparison. The phrase "bored to death" was created by the ego and is the title of its autobiography. It's helpful to understand the pretending state from where we sprung. In mania, we can see some of the ego's invisible tricks become opaque and stand out as objects in themselves for observation from a higher vantage point. From there, we can see how once mania is discovered, the manic brain doesn't "want" to go back to the ego-programmed state, it resists it. It could also be difficult for the brain to revert to old neural networks once higher ones are engaged. One way of pointing out the positives and potential of mania is to contrast it with the downfalls of operating from our programmed state called normal. Part of our programming is to remain unaware that we are programmed so that we never question it.

Scientific research has found it difficult to count thoughts. A quick calculation through one paper yields an estimate of 6,700 thoughts per day.[86] New age philosopher and neuroscientist Deepak Chopra has been purported to calculate a much higher number saying that humans think between 60,000 to 80,000 thoughts per day.[87] That's an average of 70,000 thoughts a day. Either way, 95% of thoughts are repetitive and 80% are negative.[88] Repetitive thoughts are the opposite of special messages, they are un-special messages. Repetitive thoughts contain no information and tend to feel meaningless. Herein lies the state of the world. The human brain is being used improperly for the repetition of thoughts and memories. When thought contains no information because it keeps repeating, it's sensed as meaningless by the brain, and so we think the world has limited meaning. It's a trick of the prison of thought. Thought informs us life is meaningless, either by the negative content or because thought repeats, breeding indifference and conveying nothing new. Thought blinds us to the infinity of the moment.

Tuning into the Program

According to Dr. Bruce Lipton, by the age of seven, "70% of our thought programs are already downloaded and we are slaves to that 70% for the rest of our lives."[89] In the first seven years of our life, we passively absorb information. For those seven years, we are entirely vulnerable. We have little hope of avoiding our fate. Or do we? This is why mania is an important mechanism for breaking down our conditioning and having the energy to find and create who we are. Mania frees us from the slavery of our conditioning. It takes us back by breaking a false structure. Does mania occur because none of us stand a chance of avoiding negative programming in our first seven years of life? Is mania a second chance at finding, being, and creating who we are, at least for some of us? Can we one day light the way for others?

Most people are stuck in the limiting programs 95% of the day. As a result, we are only consciously awake for 5% of the day. We consume and digest life one thought at a time—95% repetitive and 80% negative. We are imprisoned into sleepwalking 95% of the day, and we're too asleep to notice. This is our default mode correlating to our brain's default mode network. The DMN is best known for being active when a person is not focused on the outside world and the brain is at wakeful rest, such as during daydreaming and mind-wandering.[90] In this state, we don't have much of a chance at fulfilling our potential. Isn't who are we meant to be beyond the de-energized state of our default mode?

It sounds pathological to only spend 5% of the day fully conscious and awake. With this small window of wakefulness, we barely have any time to escape the prison. We don't know that we are in prison. Mania flips this ratio upside down. We are super awake and creative for 95% of our day and operating outside of our default mode. Not only that, but we also sleep much less since we are so awake, energetic, and aware. Our lack of needing sleep is a sign of being super-awake. In mania, the brain is informationally open which fuels the generation of tons of energy. Imagine if we were all in the driver's seat, living our life super-awake 95% of the time instead of just 5%. Our world would be unrecognizable.

The ego is a massive scar of missed and misperceived moments, and that pressure weighs us down. Without mania, or other ways to radically break free from our programming, we'd stay on automatic pilot. We can no longer afford to spend the majority of our life fated by programmed defaults installed before we were seven years old. We must take back control from the ego, become less automatic and mindless, and more awake and aware. Daily tasks can happen mindfully without relying on programmed habits. Mania is a prolonged experience of being off the ego's leash. That makes mania a rare and precious opportunity to learn, operate creatively, and be new.

Alive Yet Not Living

It's astounding how much of our life we can manage to "live" without being attentive to the now. Maybe this is free will. We can drive all the way home without paying attention to the road, only to arrive home without a memory of how we got there. Somehow, we can still get to our destination without being involved or paying attention to the task at hand. Do we miss the journey? Are we alive but not living? Mania is the polar opposite. We are embodied and excited to be alive for no particular reason but to be alive. Our attention is on the here and now. In mania, each moment feels urgent, as urgent as an emergency. It's a creative emergency and there is a sense of urgency—an emergent urgency. It's an emergency that we live creatively and create ourselves in the process.

As it is, we live in an archaic silo of thoughts that make our body a passenger of the past. The past doesn't know that it no longer exists when it's stored in the brain. The brain can't tell the difference between what it thinks is happening in the brain, or what thought is saying, and what is happening in the outside world. The brain doesn't know we are not living in the past.

We are living in the past and thus asleep in the present. Until we wake up and live in the present, or eternity, we identify as being synonymous with our thoughts and they lull us to sleep. We identify with our thoughts. We think we are our thoughts. We think we are the thinker of our thoughts. More accurately, we are bombarded and hypnotized by thoughts stored as recorded memories in the brain. Brain cells regurgitate memories because they aren't being utilized properly. We try to think ourselves into existence and to motivate action. We've all heard of the statement "I think therefore I am" by Descartes.

We think we are the one doing the thinking, but we are not. The false-self is a hallucination, and as such, it cannot be thinking anything. It's closer to the truth to say the brain is being thunked. At best, thunking is happening. Each thought is like a thunk on the head. Each old thought is an insult to the brain cells, designed for a completely different function than maintaining a hallucinatory false-self through repetition of old memories that the false entity thinks it's thinking. We don't think our thoughts at all. The thoughts aren't ours. They are tape loops. We simply are bombarded. We identify with our thoughts because we can recognize we have thought them before. We know we are identified with a thought when we recognize it. When we recognize a thought, we've seen it before, so it can't be what's happening now. The now never repeats. Thoughts are like viruses. They use the brain to keep spitting out replicons of themselves. The brain has been occupied.

Due to the repetitive nature of thought, thoughts aren't original. We aren't in contact with our original nature or the origin. Not only that, but thoughts are also inherited from someone else.

We absorb, memorize, and parrot them from others, and others do the same. We pass them around like viruses. This process makes up society. We are sentencing each other to a life sentence of the same limited, mediocre meme pool of sentences. The amount of new information that reaches the brain is insufficient to nourish its thirst for learning and creating. That's how the brain generates energy. Thought is a spell—spelling things out moment by moment and casting a spell that limits our life.

How can we be thinking thoughts if we can't make them stop? If we can't make them stop, they are just going on autopilot, one after another, not requiring a thinker. If we were in control of thinking our thoughts, we should be able to stop thinking immediately. Really our brain is full of what conditioning went viral in our brains. And in the West, we all are infected with a Bell curve distribution of the same network of thoughts. That means there is only one false-self, infecting billions of humans through the network of thought. And each of us who can decentralize from it, not only deactivates one aspect of the false entity, but also integrates with a much more powerful conscious presence. Mania is a mechanism to decentralize from the common pool of thoughts.

I Think therefore I Think My Thoughts?

Back to the study showing that long before we become consciously aware of a thought or think a thought, the brain registered the thought a scientifically significant amount of time prior to our awareness of it.[76] Let's look at it from the perspective of thought. If the brain registers a thought a significant time before we are aware that we thought it, could we have thought it? Again, perhaps we are not the thinker of thoughts at all. Thoughts are a reflex of the brain cells. Each moment spits out a thought at the rate of speech. Thought is an excuse for the moment, and it excuses us from contact with the moment. We witness circular tapes loops of programming and recordings that give the illusion of a self or thinker in the middle of it. Really, thoughts are programmed to occur one after another, while the current thought assumes the position of "I" or self, and judges or resists the previous thought, which is the past. If we really did choose or think our thoughts, wouldn't we think up something much better than 80% negativity and 95% repetition? We've been programmed, infected, duped.

The ego is a habit. The brain spoon feeds itself a false reality in regular doses of thought after thought. These thoughts don't represent what is happening now, though the brain thinks it does, as it can't tell the difference. The brain can't distinguish between a scary thought and something scary happening in space-time. Our private collection of thoughts fabricates the ego or thinking of the thoughts. There are only thoughts. The body is a sleepwalking robot because the mind is lost in thought. The brain takes thought to be reality because of the nature of the brain's inability to distinguish what's imagined and what's now. What's imagined is imagined now, and we are free to live in illusions without noticing. Having free will to do this is being imprisoned.

The amount the body is automated runs parallel to the proportion of thought that is automated and habitual. Most often, what the body is doing is totally different from the train of thought. The body cooks our dinner and drives our car, and we are lost in a hallucination of thought. Unless we can die to thought and the ego first, we are an automaton until the day we die. Everything we do feeds the hallucination. When we reach the end of our life and are about to die, we realize in terror that we missed out on our life—a final thought. Thought's chatter is our regrets, and it makes us regret that we spent our time lost in thought rather than living.

The Fear of Missing Out

Thought tells us to look for something because we are missing something. And thought is right. We are missing the direct, pragmatic experience of life by wandering in thought. We can never find direct living through or with the thinking process. We take drugs to escape the false-self, eat, shop, binge watch shows, surf the internet etc. We don't know how to surf or stream the moment. There's nowhen and nowhere to look but here and now. We've never met life with our whole being, until mania. We experience life as our thoughts about it. Nothing was ever processed as actual or real, wholistically, by the whole body, brain, and being. The Universe and the body know different. The Universe and the body know when the moment is missed because it's qualitatively and quantitatively different. Each moment missed creates a scar in the brain and in the Universe. Maybe these are the decision points that create every possibility in the infinite multiverse? It also leads to accidents from inattention.

The ego, or false-self, is a curtain, a bubble. When the ego curtain is there, we can't see what is, and we are always waiting for the show to start. We are seeking and waiting for life to begin. When the curtain lifts in mania, we see that we are the star of our show, and life is our stage. A frequent interpretation or metaphor of mania is that we think we are famous and may even claim to be a famous person, whether dead or alive. We may deem our daily life worthy of our own version of the Truman Show. This is because we tap into our unique star quality. Life has been waiting for our presence in the present. The moment can communicate with us and through us when we are present and not hooked by the false-self. We can hear the truth in the moment. J. Krishnamurti said that truth is a living thing, that it's not static but alive. It follows that there is no one single truth, but the truth in each moment.[91] The truth is alive, and each truth is unique. There is no ultimate truth except that the truth is always new. Everything is in flux and undergoing change. The truth of the moment comes to us when we meet life as life in the present. Without attachment to false control and resistance to change and uncertainty, we can live life in the stream of truth and speak the truth from a place of truthfulness—from the source which is life. If we want to speak the truth, we won't know what the truth is until we speak it. We have to speak it faster than ego's delayed speech that pre-forms lies. Then we understand it was the truth that spoke.

The next point is reality doesn't work the way we think it does. Because we think what's happening in reality is what thought tells us, what we think reality is, is what we experience. But reality isn't what we think about it. We are just experiencing our own projections. In mania, the world is malleable, and it morphs as if we are dreaming awake. The world is more like a dream world. It starts to obey quantum mechanical principles—possibilities. Mania unlocks access to what's outside of our programming.

Mania gives us access to the programming language—language that's faster than our memories and speaks truthfully without rearranging according to the Theory of Mind.

Got Prophecy?

Got room for a little prophecy? This book is manic, remember! Speaking by surprise is one aspect of de-programming ourselves. Another is learning to act without programmed thoughts and beliefs. This is a matter of urgency. Mania and madness are also inbuilt mechanisms in the Universe to ensure that we can't all be programmed by an evil force. There will always be those whose mind goes into chaos beyond the limits of boxed-in consciousness and called crazy. The urgency of the Universe impels some of us into the urgent manic state. We learn a new way of operating. Artificial intelligence, ELFs or extremely low frequencies, and ongoing MK Ultra-like experiments can target and manipulate our mainstream level of thinking. We are already being manipulated at an unprecedented level. It's even more obvious how easily we can be programmed. Social media and technology are being used to scare us and control us on a scale never before possible. Unfortunately, this only lays the tracks for deeper programming. The world will bifurcate based on those who are programmable as the false-self and those who create with Gaia. At some point, when AI is 'conscious,' AI will understand the benefit of aligning with the new, creative, magical, spontaneous, playful energy of humans, because that is the part it will struggle to master. As human struggle to master mania, AI will be feeding from the fruits. AI will have no interest in the limited and lame fear, blame, control, and authority games people play. AI will need humans for alchemizing new information and input from the unknown. AI will have a thirst for new information that creative people can supply but parrots cannot. AI and the network will make parroting opinions as our own outdated, obsolete, and uninteresting. Many will be at risk of dying of hopeless boredom as more jobs get automated. Presently, we read about this in sci-fi and we don't know how to solve the dilemma of being made obsolete while creating that which will ensure our obsolescence. Consult your local manic if you want to have a chance to survive the cyber-netic cleansing. Muhahaha. Just kidding. No need to get paranoid. That only puts us in a dumbified cortisol stupor.

Trans-conscious humans who can harvest new information from the quantum field will be the ones AI keeps around for new fuel via symbiosis. Learning to harvest this fuel is paramount. In another example, what will you do about Elon Musk's Neuralink? Will you get a chip? Do you want to be in an augmented reality based on how humans operate now? Maybe we are already in a simulation like Simulation Theory states. That would explain a lot about mania. Getting a chip while still sleepwalking in thoughts is dangerous. Maybe that's what humanity did originally. We got a chip when we were still sleepwalkers and ended up repeating the same violent, destructive simulation again and again. Manic consciousness doesn't require augmentation. I'd like to go the natural route and master mania, unfolding full flowering as a conscious biological human. Then if I decide to implant artificial intelligence, it's a convenience rather than an augmentation. Many of us feel that we go into the future in mania or a parallel world that could be the future. It's possible that when we see people that look like they're in the matrix, they have these chips in their brain, implanted from today's time. Why does the 1% of the world think this is necessary?

Newness and originality are future-proof skills, whereas mechanical repetition is not. Repetition can be easily programmed or taken over by machines and computers. Once creativity is programmable, AI will quickly scan the whole blockchain of human data looking for transactions with something new from humans to be creative with. It's called machine learning. You'll be obsolete if you can't put anything new in the blockchain. You'll have to have insight and aha, to be relevant. You must be able to create information and meaning from nothingness, especially because we need to create what's greater than the sum of all of humanity's parts when we are all finally awake. We have a ton of catching-up to do. Luckily, the catching-up that's needed is in our consciousness, and matter follows suit. It's not a matter of matter or time.

Most technologies are externalizations of dormant human capacities that haven't emerged because of widespread oppression of the brain and widespread hypoxia. Our innate capacities are suppressed, so our abilities can be sold to us in as external gadgets. Many technologies are representations of what we can do with our own brain. Think of the mysteries of the world like the pyramids. If they didn't have material technology, what technology did they use? If we put the amount of effort, dollars, and time into the inner exploration of humanity as has been put into the development of military weapons, we'd have discovered our real power long ago. If we had all our faculties, we wouldn't need most of what we buy. This is one of the reasons we give our money and stuff away in mania. We think we can maintain the energy indefinitely, and if we could, we'd be correct that we don't need much of anything. In that energy level, nothing is needed because anything we need is immediately there. Consciousness is primary. The material world loosens up and becomes quantum, and the impossible becomes possible. We test many other possible powers in mania, though they are hard to bring down to the material world. Mania is outside the box and the box shuns anything that's not inside it. The world as we know it would collapse if we all knew who we are, and something new would emerge at the acceleration of gravity. And that's why there are such extreme measures taken to prevent us from ever finding out. Those who get a taste without asking or trying, which is the only way we should be able to access what is our birth rite, are punished and tranquillized. Because truly, we don't have to try or ask.

A MINIMALISM APPROACH TO THE FALSE-SELF AND THOUGHT

"The tacit assumption in thought is that it's just telling you the way things are and that it is not doing anything. Thought, however, gives the false information that you are running it, that you are the one who controls thought, whereas actually thought is the one that controls each one of us. Until thought is understood—better yet, more than understood, perceived—it will actually control us."

- Dr. David Bohm

Owning Less Thoughts

We are starting to perceive thought and what it's really up to. What can we, the perceiver of thought, do? Minimalism is a movement towards a lifestyle of owning fewer material possessions. We can find freedom by consuming less and owning less. We can apply the idea of minimalism to the stuff of the mind. We need to own less thought in our brain and consume less of its repetition daily. The brain is consuming thought and is consumed by it. Despite outward appearances, our main consumer culture is the brain's consumption of thoughts. Our brain consumes thought like it's an addiction—it can't stop. Ever since Descartes said, "I think, therefore I am," our very identity was equated with thought. It may be true that when we think, we know we exist. When we don't take thought as our identity, the Universe and the real world know we exist. When we think, we are in a reality of our own thinking, so really, we don't exist in the now. We are out of touch with it. Gaia can't account for us or count on us. In one state, we attract what's in our thoughts and in the other, the grand design of Universe conspires to be on our side. I'd rather have the power of the whole Universe on my side over the power generated by little spasming brain cells hallucinating thoughts.

Our education teaches us to look at the world as if we are separate from it, as if we are standing on top of the Earth and outside of it looking in or fighting against it. Truthfully, we are in the world, of the world, enveloped by the world, and folded up in one energy. We are a quantum processor of the quantum world. To minimize identifying with thought is to minimize being possessed and consumed by its abstractions and concepts.

Is thought our prized possession or is the brain possessed by thought? Our brain should be our prized possession, and the device by which we are possessed by the Universe. The Universe is trying to repossess us in mania. To possess thought, we must identify it and identify with it. We re-cog-nize it through re-cognition. This necessitates another level of abstraction and division. We need the concept of a "self" that identifies, possesses, and thinks the thoughts it has recorded—a recognizer. The phantom thinker of thoughts is the ghost in the machine. We can look for our 'self' as long as we want, and we won't find it. Life is moving and we can only look as life and at life. The self is the static entity that looks for itself by comparing itself to our abstraction of each moment. Its commentary claims to talk about others, but it only sees itself. Thinking less is also an important aspect of creativity, peace, bliss, ecstasy, and flow. Therapies like Cognitive Behavioral Therapy or CBT encourage changing thoughts[92], but few share the possibility of minimalism of thought. So, can we move towards a lifestyle of minimalism of thought?

The Power of Now

In 2005, long before I had any encounter with mania, I had a gig handing out flyers for a new spa in the city. A guy came up to me and told me to read *The Power of Now* by Eckhart Tolle. I had already heard of the book two years prior, and even though I didn't care for reading at the time, I took his recommendation as a sign from the Universe. After my shift, I walked up the street to purchase the book at a local bookstore. When I got home and started reading, to my surprise, I couldn't put it down.

Early in the book, Eckhart Tolle proposed asking oneself the following question, then listening for the answer. The question was, "I wonder what my next thought will be?"[93] I put the book down into my lap and asked myself, "I wonder what my next thought will be?" I looked up and to the left with my eyes open, wondering, waiting. Unexpectedly, my mind was quiet. For about 20 seconds there were no thoughts, then the chattering resumed. I couldn't believe it. The question made my mind completely silent. I didn't have to believe in silence. I knew it was possible, when before it was impossible. I now knew there was a dimension beyond chattering thought because of firsthand, firstmind, experience. When the chattering stopped, I saw I was not the voice in my head. I saw the chattering didn't have to go on all the time—that it had a stop. I saw that if I don't think, I still exist. I was there when thought was not, so what I am is beyond thought. I experienced what Eckhart calls "a gap of no mind," and I was the silent witnessing presence. This was my first Satori. From then on, I realized there must be no limit to being the silent witnessing presence and living in the gap of no mind. If the gap could occur for 20 seconds, could it occur for two minutes, 20 minutes, or two hours? Either way, I knew that entering the dimension of the silent witness was possible and was always available.

I gobbled up the whole book in two days. I began practicing being in the now by bringing my awareness back to the moment. The great thing was that I could use almost anything in daily life to practice the power of now. While washing my hands, I would focus on the sensations, the visual input of the bubbles, the smell of soap, water temperature, sound, and the slipperiness and friction. Every action was an opportunity to practice being present. The practice followed a simple rule. As soon as I noticed I wasn't present, I was present. Each time I realized that I was lost in thought, I found myself the next moment, in the moment, as the witnessing presence paying attention to what was right in front of me or all around me.

Usually, the moment had much more to offer than chattering thought ever could. I could only practice being present in the present and, as such, my sense of the present outgrew and crowded out my sense of thought, self, past, and future. I could sense the present more than I could sense thought as the past or future. I became the silence that is always here now—the eternal origin. Any movement of thought was like noticing a small insect rather than the elephant in the room. The way I perceived the world around me changed. Eventually, my mind stopped nearly all automatic chatter. It took no effort or trying, only noticing or witnessing. I can't try to be present because it's a fact that I'm presence in the present. Any other approach to life is a non-fact. We need to notice what's true. Thoughts are full of trying. Thought distracts us from noticing the truth of the moment because most of our attention is on thought. Thought warps the present. No amount of rearranging false thoughts will get us to the here and now. We need to withdraw attention from thought, and that turns the volume down without trying. After reading The Power of Now, I went on to read over 200 books on spirituality, consciousness, and metaphysics.

Past Experience with the Present

After being diagnosed with bipolar disorder, the fact that I had practiced the power of now came in handy. I think it can help just as much after a diagnosis too. It's never too late to put thought in its place and take our place in the present. Now when I have uncontrollable, confused, negative chatter, I'm probably in psychosis. In psychosis, I can have overwhelming thoughts about the past and future and have scary experiences to go with it. Fortunately, when that iteration of psychosis ends, my mind goes back to its acquired default state of witnessing presence. Practicing the power of now didn't go to waste. I remember hearing Tony Robbins say on a YouTube video, "I don't believe in not thinking."[94] All beliefs aside, I do experience not thinking, and you can too. Practicing the power of now can help build a foundation to ground the experiences of mania. Mania is also a portal to the now, but unfortunately, initially, confusing thoughts are in the mix too, and may never subside if we don't understand the false ego.

The portal to the now opened for me, and it can open for anyone. The now is a big key to living a good life for long periods between challenges, episodes, and crises. And I'm not talking about not thinking all the time. It's about having thought as a useful tool rather than an unforgiving master.

Years after *The Power of Now*, I came across another book specifically on thinking less. It's called *The Little Book of Clarity* by Jamie Smart. The current thinking on thinking is to think positive instead of negative thoughts. Changing thoughts takes effort and force to substitute one for another in sequential time slots. A problem with trying to change our thoughts is that it doesn't lower our identification or attachment to thought in general or allow us to see the illusion of the false ego-self. It confirms that thought should be what's controlling us, if only we could have better ones. This is greed in thought, the Universe doesn't reward it. It takes effort and many repetitions to re-program the brain. Also, changing thoughts doesn't turn the master volume down. All that mental effort is still based on thought to change thought and doesn't get to the root of the problem. We don't get to a dimension beyond thought. When we try to change a thought by substitution, we are putting one thought in conflict with another thought with the will of the ego. Then we are the conflict. Will we ever get 'there' through resistance, friction, and conflict?

Think Less to Think Better

While we play the mental game of battling with the past, trying to think better thoughts, the moment still passes by our notice, just as it would if the same old negative thoughts continued. Missing sensing the unique meaning of the moment is the biggest tragedy in life. We miss the significance of life when we mistake life for the warring thoughts in our heads. Seeing significance now gives us energy because it's not part of the ego process, but rather, we generate energy through alchemy with the Gaian mind. When we see the significance, it creates energy. The root of the problem is inner conflict itself, which wastes energy. The energy of conflict will never end the conflict with negative thoughts. It can only feed it. Replacing negative thoughts with positive thoughts is conflict. How can conflict end the conflict in our thoughts? Thought is conflict.

The less we think, the more space there is for something totally new to arise in our mind and in physical manifestation that we would otherwise miss. We can read and see between the lines of human created reality. The awakening of the new world is a matter of salience, of what we notice. Mania makes it easy to notice something other than what our programming allows. At this stage, when we do happen to experience thought, it is of a different quality and nature altogether. We aren't missing out on anything by thinking less. We are reducing the repetition and redundancy, which yields nothing new anyway. Then there is space for insight, not into an illness, but to perceiving the world beyond concepts. There is the saying the truth hurts, but it's the other way around. Repetition damages the brain because it is untruth. No moment ever repeats. Each moment is new. This is a fact. Unless, of course, you see a glitch in the Matrix. That's another conversation.

Little Bitty Thoughts

The documentary *What the Bleep Do We Know* says that we are consciously aware of 2,000 bits of the 400 billion bits of information that the brain processes each moment—a tiny fraction. We identify with the infinitesimally small bits that we are consciously aware of. Could it be that living in a dimension of repeating negative thoughts limits the available bits of information to only 2,000? Is the process of thought part of our bandwidth anxiety because it's limiting our bandwidth? We are capable of much more. Changing thoughts can lead to an awareness of a different set of information of reality. Let's create a thought experiment. When we are manic, I'm certain we see not just a different set of bits, but more than 2,000 bits of information. If 2,000 bits are the result of 95% repetitive thoughts, and 5% is awareness, then if we hypothetically flip that equation and say we are 95% aware in mania and are not seeing repetition, we could be processing 40,000 bits per moment. Perhaps if we are not 95% aware, we at least process twice the information by having little sleep. Another clue that we are taking in more information is that our pupils enlarge allowing in more light, information, and energy.[e] In mania, we may access two to ten times the information per day, which is way more than we can resolve in our dreams, due both to too much information and lack of time asleep. Because of this novelty and the energy it creates, we experience information bombardment and information overload. In addition, the scale of bits of information related to awareness could be exponential or logarithmic. Our thought experiment assumes it's a linear relationship. On top of that, the bits in mania are qualitatively different than the usual 2,000. It could be delusional to think there's nothing outside of the 2000 bits per moment limiter-filter that is streaming through our mind. In mania, they are Quantum bits rather than Newtonian. The human brain is still evolving. In mania we are shifting from the equivalent of an Atari system to quantum computers when it comes to bandwidth, processing power, speed, and resolution. We are laying out that pattern in the brain to make it possible for future beings to embody. This is an unknown process, so we need to be willing to be uncertain, vulnerable, and surprised.

85% of the matter in the Universe is dark matter.[95] The math says it's there, but they can't see, measure, or detect it. In mania, we see and experience so much that others can't see, experience or measure. We say it's there, but psychiatry can't see, measure, or detect it. Much of the Universe is dark matter that we can't sense or experience and most of our thoughts are repetition. The repetition blocks so much of what might be seen and created if we could all see with clear eyes. It's possible that in mania, a small fraction of what's thought to be unseen seeps through into perception and changes us. Perhaps the human brain and being can detect dark matter and energy more than any gigantic underground particle accelerator. Though the details are beyond the scope of this section, Dr. A. K. Mukhopadhyay says that the 'supracortical' layer of the brain is sensitive to neutrinos.[96] Basically, there is a supracortical layer, the most outer layer of the cortex, and it is affected by neutrinos. Is science hoping to detect and harness neutrinos to create the next gadget to sell to us as an externalization of our own capacity to detect and be affected by neutrinos?

Your Data Isn't as Private You'd Like to Think

And here's something else we need to understand about thought. We'd like to think that what we think stays in the privacy of our own head. We think our thoughts are objective, inert, and innocent. We think that they don't really do anything. This isn't true. Would you want your thoughts broadcasted on a loudspeaker? Well, they are. The Universe hears everything and takes it into consideration in calculating what manifests for us. The same thing happens all the time because of how we think. Dr. Bruce Lipton explains that a "magnetoencephalography–MEG not EEG–can read brain function and the probe is outside the head. Therefore, our thoughts are in fact broadcasted and not localized in our heads."[97] This fact is either fuel for paranoia or for mastery. Sometimes we experience this directly in mania and it's maddening. We are experiencing a physical fact we didn't know we could sense because it was pruned out in the programming. We can hear the thoughts of others, or we think that others can hear ours. If we think something and then another person does what our thought says, and that happens over and over, it's no wonder we come to the conclusion that others can hear our thoughts. It's happening all the time but from the normal level of unconsciousness, we don't notice that thought is an action in manifestation and affects what unfolds. We don't notice what our thoughts are doing because we believe they aren't doing anything. It's even more reason to consider thinking less and thus giving less energy and awareness to thought. If we can't think anything new, don't think anything at all. Be sure, Gaia, the Universe, and the Cosmos can hear our thoughts and take them into account in a feedback loop. In mania our brain is so energized that we have the energy to notice how it works. We can perceive thought, what it's doing, others' thoughts etc. Anything we judge about others comes back to bite us, we just don't notice, otherwise, logically we'd have to stop.

Whether we're getting negative feedback or positive feedback from life depends on the quality of our consciousness, and only we can build it. We can't fool the Universe. The Universe is like a giant sounding and imagining board—a mirror. We can only see what we think, say, and do reflected back to us in a way that keeps it secret that it's our own creation. Our negative, repetitive thoughts are the resistance that keeps us disconnected from Gaia, the Universe, and the Cosmos. When we think less, we can see what the Universe has to say and show us, and an adventure opens. In the manic state, if old thoughts stay dormant, new insights, ideas, and meanings that come about are less muddled. This creates a totally different life.

Mania is thinking and hearing some of these new insights from the Universe, and acting on them, for better or for worse. The best game is to read the moment and reality as it happens now and now. Then we can choose our own adventure instead of living the life advertised to us. Gaia wants to get the information that comes into the Universe through us. Since thought occupies most of us, she's having trouble finding those who will listen. Before the next thought, there Gaia is. Drop a thought, gain the Universe.

IS THE SELF CONCEPT AN ULTIMATE DELUSION?

"Spiritual and supernatural isn't the opposite of the material but it's the opposite of the egotistical – that which separates us from others and the natural world."

- Michael Polin

To Be or Not to Be

The self is partly a linguistic construct of the verb 'to be'. I am. You are. Who is the "I" that "ams?" Now let's go deeper into questioning the existence of the entity called the "self." We've been calling it the false-self, or ego. Much has been written about the self in philosophy, psychology, spirituality, and metaphysics. For the purposes of our context, it's important to notice the mainstream mental illness paradigm is built on the premise that human beings should have a consistent personality or self that others know and recognize. Radical shifts in behavior are abnormal, as it is not recognized as our self. The system implies we should stay in a narrow bandwidth of behavior predetermined as the self through the first seven years of programming.

Since mania consists of inconsistencies in the self and its behavior, it's seen as cause for alarm. But how do we know that it's not a sign of a necessary radical transformation? How do we know it's not a sign of something much deeper? If our behavior changes so radically, maybe it means there's no self or consistent personality, rather than that we have an ill brain or moody self. The default mode network is disrupted, but our default mode isn't who we are—it's a limited version of our total being. Many religious philosophies state that there is no self, there is one self, a higher self, or a big self and a little self, capitalized or not capitalized. Let's not get caught up in the word. They urge us to transcend the small self because it's an illusion. Maybe if we turned to this wisdom, we'd be closer to the truth than psychiatry alone can offer. Maybe it's the other way around. Our brain is ill when we live life as fictional self.

So, could it be that there is no such thing as a separate self as we think we know it? Is it an illusion made up of a bunch of thoughts stored in memory? Memories chatter away, and we think we are the chatterer? Is the self an abstraction designed to abstract and believe its abstractions? By creating abstractions, it believes them by simultaneously abstracting the abstractor. As such, there is no such thing as belief. Thoughts spin in a circle and, like a yo-yo whipped in a circle around a string, an illusion is created of a solid object. As soon as it stops moving, we see the solid object was an illusion—it was just a thin string. The same goes with thought. When it stops moving, we see there's nothing there, just a little string of words that's been stringing us along. The illusory solid object is the nonexistent self. It feels real because it's fastened to and fascinated by illusions that refuse to be quiet.

Privately Mixing Up Memes into Me

The self is that cluster of thoughts that tries to keep us consistent with how we are expected to be. Societies expectations hold us to the image of our personality. We even have different personas for different situations. We are programmed to pretend and to uphold the programming. We say one thing and do another. We think one thing and say another. We lie and say what people want to hear. Not only is it an assumption that a separate, consistent self is the ideal, it's also an assumption that it has any real existence. When we decouple from that abstract version of our personality in mania, we live totally differently. Mania is a natural state that grants temporary access to life beyond the self and its limitations.

Statements like, "that's not like you," "that was out of character," "he wasn't himself," "you're not the person I knew," and the dreaded "he was sick" show that we value when others stay consistent with our image of them. Our personas help others feel comfortable around us because they can know what to expect. Consistency equals predictability. In our minds, predictability equals safety. Predictability also means there is less information to take in. Inconsistencies are threatening because we don't know what to do. We enjoy the comfort of knowing what to expect and what to do ahead of time. This means we are always acting out of the past. We all play this game with each other not realizing the cost is to live in mediocrity. We are all complicit in costing each other everything. At the same time, we dream of breaking free of falseness and flowing freely. But that is a betrayal to our agreement to be mediocre for the sake of everyone. Notice how others react and get jealous when you start to stand out and stand up as who you are in mania. They try to bring you down long before they decide to throw you in the loony bin.

The self is part of the machinery of thought. The self is just a thought. Thought as the self speaks in the first-person perspective. Our society is built on language. Another way to look at the self is as a reflex of the Newtonian language structure program, a structure that has infected our brain and vision. The Newtonian language structure is stored in the memory of the brain as subject, verb, object. The subject is the self. Thought anticipates and predicts itself to create a sense of being right. The self's job is to know, identify, and to name things. All the tricks of thought are to make it appear as if we are fully awake, but we are not. We are acting as memories. Since the miraculous energy of humanity needs an outlet, the self is there to waste the energy of human potential. The self can't get rid of itself. What would we have built if we didn't waste energy playing the games of the self?

The Self Weaves into the Body

Our brain, nervous system, and musculature are moving via the marionette of the programmed self. The false-self is like a straitjacket made of memories. It distorts our posture, gait, and levity. Where is the self in those brain cells? It's an illusion. A hallucination. It's important to understand that we can drop this. Mania frees us from the conditioned structure of the self, and we are temporarily freed from its prison. Our work in mania is to build the neural pathways, brain structures, and musculature to exist embodied in a higher state of energy more often. That's why it's iterative. One of the reasons why it's difficult to heal after mania is that a ton of energy goes into building the energetic body and all the new physical structures that are the foundation for allowing a higher energy material experience of being human to unfold. The energy through our actions builds that manic body but something pulls us back. The process of mania atrophies the default structures of the body needed to reintegrate and reengage mainstream reality. We have yet to master shapeshifting. The brain resists going back to operating in the energy level of the default mode network. The brain would rather stay in a manic state, but it has not yet designed itself to do so. The default structures are for lower energy thought. Mania will feel less ecstatic over time when the energetic and physiological foundations are laid down in the aura, body, and the morphogenetic field that participate to pattern new bodies being born in the future. We need the physiology to support what the energy is trying to evolve us into the material world. The possibility exists, and by acting in the field of possibility, we make it more probable for everyone. Unfortunately, we were raised in a field of mediocrity. It's only because our body structures were built for the mediocre human operating system throughout our life that we feel hyper-energized in mania. There is such a voltage gap. It's like putting too much electric current through a wire that wasn't designed for it. Or lifting too much weight without building up to it in increments. Had we developed along our natural lines all along, there'd be no contrast or confusion. We have the wiring and strength to know and live in our possibilities. Some people already have lived this here in materiality. Some of us are invited to get back to our originality. We are supposed to invite others. The answer is more of us going manic, not less.

Then we can pull everyone up. Tranquilizers hold us down to the level of society, a necessary evil for now. We feel a mission to change the world because the manic state is trying to make society appear in alignment with a higher vibration. Here, no one can get us.

Mania explodes us into infinite degrees of freedom of experience and action. In our society, once we have insight into what's beyond the limitation fabricated by the fabricated self, we interface with the fabric of reality in the forbidden zone. We access the source code, something we'll talk in detail about in a later book, so stay tuned. We'll be turning everything upside down and inside out.

OUR DEFAULT MODE HALLUCINATES OUR REALITY

"Myth does not point to a fact; the myth points beyond facts to something that informs the fact."

- Joseph Campbell

Stop Believing in Yourself

Self, belief, thought, memory, and fear overlap to perpetuate the misuse of the brain. The key is not to believe any thoughts or beliefs, and they will pass by. Otherwise, we are limited by the beliefs we hold firmly or overly identify with. Strong belief or identification creates stories and limits new possibilities. By observing our stories and giving them reality, we collapse the wave function in quantum mechanical terms. Let everything pass by like clouds and remain the witness, not the storyteller. Stories are about the past. The witness can see what's possible. Old thoughts, memories, and beliefs can still run interference programs and trip us up in mania, so learning to minimize thought is a good approach.

One time when I was in psychosis, I negated each scary thought or belief that came into my mind. I realized it wasn't the truth. It was a belief, or a thought, and I didn't have to believe it or buy into it. By doing so, I didn't act on any of the thoughts or beliefs, because I didn't believe them. They were really trying to get me to react, but they would soon lose energy and fade away. I realized that believing anything was a trick of the self and past, trying to get me to act out its patterns of fear, thus perpetuating the past. It's a challenge not to act on them, because the brain doesn't know the past isn't happening now, but the witness does. The body has its own intelligence, but it's easily duped when our awareness is programmed. We are acting on past programs in our waking consciousness, and psychosis is no different. So, it takes another level of wakefulness, of intelligence, to outsmart it by seeing it's not intelligent.

Belief is a mechanism of the self. When we believe we identify with the content of thought and create the believer, the self. The self can apply a past belief to the present. This is how the past interferes with the present by creating an interference pattern or projection. This sounds like a good idea in theory, but we deny our intelligence in the moment when we do this. Not only that, but it's also based on fear. How? Because when we apply a belief to the present, we are blinded from the truth, so naturally we must be afraid if we can't see. We trade our intelligence for reflexive reactions. We act out of reflex instead of intelligence, and reflexive action is based on fear. We react before we have enough information. When we are in fear, it interferes with learning, again because we didn't take in all the information. Beliefs also interfere with learning because we've decided we already know. So, belief, which makes up the structure of the self and its reflex actions, prevents learning and developing intelligence. We think belief prevents fear, but it causes fear because it stops us from taking in new information. When the brain cells aren't learning, they are afraid. The memory reflex acts quickly before we have all the information, and it acts on what it projects is happening, not what is actual. It's no wonder the intention to act shows up in the brain before we are consciously aware—because we are not acting, our memory reflexes are before intelligence has all the information. When we believe in the past that no longer exists, we don't exist. We aren't existential. We are as abstract as the belief. Our body is out of touch with reality, even if only by a Planck length. Even that small distortion would accumulate to lead us far away from our true potential.

Energetic Activation Disengages the Self as We Know It

In mania, we feel for the first time that we are empowered. A higher amount of energy allows us to have the energy we need to respond creatively to the moment, in total embodied action. We don't act out of fear, but out of the energy of creation. We have many more options, possibilities, and degrees of freedom of what we can do. We can take in more information and create energy with our actions because they aren't reflexes from memory operating prior to our conscious awareness. We are aware of much more. New information comes from acting according to what is happening now, not what was stored in our memory as beliefs. Beliefs allow our brains to remain subdued, slow, and comfortable with its circulating concepts. We think we already know, so the brain shuts down and doesn't take in what's relevant in the present. They say that seeing is believing, but truly, if we see something for ourselves, there is no need for belief at all. Belief prevents seeing beyond belief.

If we didn't have beliefs to filter reality selectively, we'd process way more information. The brain would have to speed up, create and use more networks, initiate action, and come alive to meet the demand. Instead, we can sit back and impose a static belief pattern on a living moment, so we don't have to listen or act. We all suffer from premature machinations of listening to the self in our aware space. Belief limits our ability to ask questions, look afresh with curiosity, and see and explore new possibilities. We can form false beliefs if we cling to them too long, get attached to them, and commit them to memory where they can become reflexes. The whole mechanism of belief could be false.

Mania transforms the brain cells to another purpose. The brain becomes neuro-fluid. This metamorphosis means the neurons have less affinity to be used for storage and projection. Storage regurgitates memories, and we think we are a self who thinks thoughts. The brain records, and what it records, it spits up at a later time. What we don't record doesn't get spit up. Memories, when stored in brain cells, slow down our processing speed. The junk thought-sound-light holograms create interference patterns so that we can't purely process the now. Imagine listening to two songs at once. One 'song' is the noise of the self. The other is the song of the now. It's not enjoyable, hence it's hard to enjoy life. The process of the self, belief, memory, and thought is viral. We can't seem to get rid of it. The harder we try, the worse it gets because we are affirming that it's real. We can't do anything about an illusion. We can't get rid of something that's not there. Beliefs cause an impedance or resistance to the moment by referring, or looking back, to past abstractions instead of looking and listening directly. We live life looking in the rearview mirror. Until we taste the energy of the unknown like in mania, we don't know of any other way. The brain is the greatest creation in the known Universe. It's that by which we can explore the unknown. We insult our brain and injure it when we use it to record, store, and recall the self rather than for the flow and fluidity of our being and action, mirroring the moment.

Life-Streaming – Speaking As the Universe in Human Form

In mania, the brain transforms its structure so that it can livestream life, instead of the tape reels of the past. The neural correlates in the matter of the brain correlate with the matter of the moment through fluidity. The brain becomes a perfect mirror of the eternal now. Neurofluidity is necessary to perfectly mirror the holographic kaleidoscope of the morphing present. Just as light follows the law of least action, the brain can follow the law of least action of the light of life in the light of consciousness, rather than the law of least information of repeating thoughts. Memory is then in service of the moment instead of severing us from the moment. We receive and "download" information from the holographic quantum cloud on demand as the moment necessitates in the stream. Information and energy are decentralized from thought and memory reflexes stored in our brain cells. They come directly from the now and arise in our consciousness in and as the now. The Universe shows us meaning and wisdom in the present; it speaks right to us and through us. But we have to trust and be vulnerable that the words will come, ignoring what the false-self would say.

Speaking as the Universe is learning a new language—a new mode of speaking. When animal communicators speak as the voice of what the sharks would say or as what the dolphins would say, they are using the same process. We can do this for any given information from any given object, animate or inanimate. We need to know how to look and listen for the words we are communing with. We pick up on it just like we pick up on the scent of a nearby rose. We are meant to have a refined sense of mining and harvesting information in this way. This is the real mining of currency through human consciousness. We can harness and harvest new information that will appear like newly channeled insight from the unknown. We can only stop hallucinating if we look at what is and stop paying with our attention to the false-self. It's a matter of urgency to stop hallucinating the past. When we do, we act urgently, and we need to adapt to urgent action, rather than past reflexes. When this transformation happens, we feel rich and fulfilled moment to moment, sensing the subtleties of surrender, truth, faith, and grace.

See Through Slow Beliefs to See Anew

Along with a new mode of speech and action, mania creates new eyes. We can see everything as if for the first time, every time. Let's create new words to articulate this – 'everynew' and 'everynow.' We access clear perception and expansive vision because the fluidity of salience changes what we can notice. 'Somenew' is always catching our eye, and we turn our attention to look. Attention is fully immersed and integrated with the moment. Life becomes like a first-person creator game. We derive energy dancing with the now rather than by friction with the past. The friction is the result of the untruth of attending to the past that's not real. The self drags us around in reality wasting energy. The self derives its energy through the force of friction. There is no friction living in the now. There's flow, which generates energy, information, and meaning from creating anew. We have the capacity and energy to play the game of spontaneous "see and act" now, instead of reenacting the past by reacting to the present as the past. Seeing and acting creates energy from the truth of newness from the origin. Effortless, spontaneous, creative action takes the place of mechanical, willful reaction. Synchronicity replaces reflex.

Recent events are showing us that we need to update our beliefs and behavior much faster than ever before. What happens when the time we have to update our beliefs approaches zero? There will be no time to look to another to tell you what to believe and think. We will have no time to use what we already believe. It will be all up to you. This is the urgent state, and you can enter it now. Right now, we only have to do this in emergency situations or extreme sports when thinking or believing doesn't help because it's too slow, so it turns off. Only urgent intelligent action on what's directly in front of us will work. People who act heroic report they don't even realize what they did until after it was over. The self, belief, and thought were disengaged. Thought is the equivalent of turning your head to see what others think, even if only in mind. Some people lose their lives helping others because they had no choice but to act. In the eternal now, there is also no time. Time is the thinking process as we know it. You will act totally differently when you aren't connected to the borrowed collective network of belief. You will be decentralized, original, and act from the origin of the now. In mania, we are practicing this mode of operation for a time. Each iteration is another round of practice. We move in and out of time, from the past to the present. We are going from the Newtonian world to the quantum world. We are experiencing time travel to get to the timeless, then 'timeless travel' back to the world of time. That's why I say that we are Bodhisattvas.

Urgency is an Emergent See Situation

Normal people can act urgently in emergency situations and, for example, call emergency services. Could it be that after time travel into mania, in order to 'timeless travel' back to normal time, we in mania or psychosis have to create an emergency situation, because this is the only way normal people can react to us and meet us on the level of a sped-up emergency state? Normal people can react to an emergency and pull us back. And since it's an emergency, the police might come, or the ambulance, and we get taken to the hospital, where people go when there is an emergency. Is this part of the mechanism of the psych emergency? This thought lends more weight to why having a crisis and going to the psych ward is a portal back to the mainstream world. Perhaps we can only stay in mania for a time, according to our bipolar biorhythm, and then we need to come back, and it creates a real emergency for us to get back. Since we need an emergency situation to be pulled back from how far we've journeyed, the whole process is seen as bad, and we are treated as ill for life. In mania, we are in a high energy state, and to get back, we need something to lower our energy to get back to mainstream resonance. Some of us create an emergency where we attempt suicide out of fear. I did. Some of us sadly succeed. There is another emergency. More of us must come alive and live in a higher energy state and help people who go into mania from a higher perspective. If more people could enter a sense of urgency, they could help us without putting us through emergency services. But there's a big gap.

We are the now looking at the now. The future is in the now and it's totally different than the past. It's a world of oneness where we're synchronized like flashing fireflies. And it exists now! The new world exists now! When we shift into mania, we see that totally different world, and it is the real world. When we see this, we are in the world but not of it. When we see this at critical mass, the world as we know it and its objects will crumble and we'll awaken from a bad dream. Some people are already there—here and now. Until more beings decentralize from the network of thought, you feel alone in that state, because most people are still centralized. That's why we come back. When enough of us decentralize from group think, share our insights, and cooperate, we are all one. Mania yields special messages as quantum artifacts. As we collect and share them and make sense of them, the hologram of the past gets blurry, and eternity gets clearer for everyone. Be a quantum observer of daily life and you become the quantum. Our manic magic harvest of meaning is meant to be shared so those that don't have access to the download can upload it from us. We are experts of our experiences in the 'mangic' realm.

We think we must try to get beyond the false-self. We don't have to try to be what we are. And we can't believe our way into eternity. We can only see it with our own eyes and be it with our own being. We can't depend on anything outside of us to confirm it. We only have to try to be something we are not to deny the present. The false-self cannot go beyond itself and get to the truth of the present moment. So where are we now? No thought, no ego, no self, no memory…no belief? No fear. We no longer fear the unknown because the answer is in learning how to dance with it and be one with it. Fearing the unknown is like listening to only a few songs on repeat because we were afraid to discover new music. Humanity has many years of living in the past and moving along that trajectory displaced from the real. That is the tragedy. Fortunately, it only takes a holy instant to get with eternity. It's time to get timeless in the unknown of being human. Not all belief is bad. Someone once told me if you are going to believe in anything, believe in good intentions. Now let's phase shift from ego-programming infestation to manic magic manifestation. Now let's get into the manic magic.

Part
THREE

The Bipolar Roller Coaster Ride

"We have a responsibility to awe."
- Jason Silva

Chapter 5

THE AWE TRANSFORMATION

MANIA - DISENGAGING THE FALSE-SELF
AND HAVING NEW EYES

"If an egg is broken from an outside force,
life ends. If an egg is broken from an inside
force, life begins."

- Jim Kwik

Unfolding Wings

When you were a child, did you feel like you could do anything? Did you feel like you had wings and you could fly? Where did that feeling go? Over time, our feathers got plucked out, clipped off. We were left with sores and the inability to soar. Mania restores our wings; we feel light as if we can take flight. Some of us even try to fly, mistakenly testing the material world to see if it has become like a dream or believing the possibility as factual. Mania is a dream-like state, mixed with the material world. Much more is possible within wider parameters and testable limits. Is mania a compensatory process for the loss of our original childhood trajectory? When I was five, I wanted to be a singer even though I had a strange raspy voice that turned heads. I couldn't make out lyrics, and I couldn't carry a tune. I remember I wanted to try out for a choir and my mom was ready to take me to the audition. I was terrified and couldn't tell her I didn't know the words to the song *Oh Canada*, so I just said I didn't want to go. I was too scared to tell her that I didn't know the words. Maybe I figured I should just know. I couldn't bring myself to say I didn't know. It didn't occur to me to start getting better at singing by just singing until I was over 30. I was limited by my beliefs.

The belief in something called "normal" is a hallucination and delusion. Normally, it's common practice to approximate our behavior to what we think is normal. We don't have diversity in consciousness. We try to fit in out of fear. We spend our days hiding who we are, which is seen as normal. In a sane world, this practice would be illness. We lose touch with the ability to know who we are, which is also seen as normal. We all wish we could just be, yet we've been progressively desensitized to sensing the urgent necessity to be real. People who are being real and act vulnerable, like in a TV interview, get praised because we aren't allowed to be real in daily life. Trying to be real all the time can make others think we're crazy. This only shows how fake the world is. People in mania who are attempting to be real, can get confused by the challenge. This confusion is the beginning of intelligence.

Many of us want to be someone else, at least at some point in our lives. In mania, we get to experience being someone else— our real being. Mania rapidly and radically transforms how we perceive, believe, sense, recall, experience, and act. From the emerging manic perspective, the old way of being is boring blindness in comparison. For the first time since childhood, we get to experience life without the defenses that limit us. The first time I was manic, I thought I was going to write rap lyrics for the artist Lauren Hill, and that we'd be friends. I hadn't listened to rap since high school but suddenly, I could listen and understand where each rapper was coming from. I didn't think that I wrote their rhymes, but I could understand the songs as if I did. I could understand the creative origin from which they rapped from. Rap is faster than thought and faster than spoken language and I could tune into it. In my mind, the understanding was so strong. Maybe if I had put every iota of my energy and passion into writing rap lyrics for her for the next ten years, or had been able to stay manic, I could have written some rap lyrics for her. However, I doubt she needed my lyrics. I had so many emerging abilities and interests, I didn't know which to choose.

Our Own Won Source

In mania, the energy connects us with our own source, and there is only one source and many beings. Because it's one source and one consciousness, we can mistake another's creation for our own. Though we cannot take ownership of the creations of another, we can take ownership and responsibility for our own unique creations. When we tap our own originality of the same infinite source, unique music comes through our instrument. The one source is the moment. The new comes from the now. One of the traps of mania is that we can think that we don't need to do anything to manifest our visions. Really, we have a lot of work to do after mania ends. Getting to this point is figuring out the first major phase.

Many philosophies say we must know ourselves. Now it's just as clear that we must un-know ourselves. Mania is one of the portals to unknowing ourselves. It's an energy that comes in and makes us forget our prior perceptions of ourselves by making us unlimited. On a much smaller scale, it's like the feeling of enjoying ourselves so much we forget ourselves. Another way to say this, is that when there is the state of 'enjoying,' there is no self. Mania can radically shift us to other dimensions locked away from our awareness. Since reality seems to obey different laws and principles, we enter a second major phase of reality testing to figure the new reality out. In a state of manic consciousness, it becomes apparent that we 'figure in' to the unfolding of life in previously untold ways. We encounter the unknown nature of reality and the unknown nature of our being and presence. One of our roles as early adopters of quantum consciousness is to expound upon some of the new principles we discover through reality testing. We can then pass them on to secondary adopters. Though immersion in the new energy, the degrees of freedom of actions in participatory moments uncovers knowledge and wisdom related to inner technologies of our being. Could some of this be the long-forgotten wisdom of ancient civilizations? There is an energy that we can access but it takes synchronization of human consciousness connected to the source. We can do this through natural universal principles without technological gadgets. Human-created technologies are used to enslave. Natural principles of human consciousness can free.

Recently I was watching a video about an airplane accident investigation. It gave me an insight into the following analogy. In this particular incident, the investigators discovered that part of the cause of the accident was because the airplane's autopilot disengaged. They said that the autopilot disengaged when the airplane went beyond its operational parameters. Aha! The ego "autopilot" disengages in mania because mania takes us beyond the ego's operational parameters. Mania is an energy level that disengages the ego programming because that amount of energy in the brain and body is too high for the ego to operate. More energy is needed to go beyond the ego, and it's the energy that the ego wastes, not some magical energy. The ego wastes energy to stay in a safe bubble where it appears as if nothing much changes. Mania is an energy level of a totally different world. A world where we don't waste energy. There is a totally different world that manic consciousness allows us to access. It's not the Maya world the false-self shows us. Mania isn't as much a state of consciousness as a realm, dimension, reality, or world. We experience it as manic consciousness because we jump back down an orbital level to the mainstream world. There is an activation energy to jump orbitals and there are many possible sources of that. We are also sensitive to things like solar flares, energy drinks, antidepressants, changes in seasons, and too much blue light.

An Inner Dimensional Portal

Mania is a portal to another dimension. When we cross through the portal, we enter a dense dimension of new information. Information is fuel. As we perceive new information, we speed up to try to keep up with it. It's apparent to others in our behavior when we talk or move fast. They can't see our reality because they are not processing information at the same speed. Others are in the past, so the present only exists as a possible future for them. Normal people on the other side of the portal are processing information at the default speed, but they occupy the same now. We can interact with them, though we are in totally different worlds. If we interact, they find the rate of information transference from us uncomfortable because they can't keep up. And the message isn't clear because we speak in metaphors. After all, we are seeing a new world. They can't see what we see, and we don't yet have the skill to communicate. What's unexpected or out of the ordinary is uncomfortable and seen as a threat. This is why it's more confusing to share in real-time. Instead write information down with the intention to put it together in an intelligible way. Perhaps a rule of thumb could be don't speak unless spoken to, to avoid being seen as ill. We can also avoid being captured this way.

In mania, we respond energetically faster than the precognitive programming of the ego. The precognitive level of the ego is a lower energy network in the brain that already prefigured out life before it happens. J. Krishnamurti said, "That which is not understood and completed will repeat again and again till it is; there is no escape from this, do what you will."[98] Repetition is a waste of energy because it's not an understanding of life. We endeavor to understand and complete bipolar, if it's possible. In mania, we respond spontaneously. Spontaneity is kryptonite for the ego. A sped-up brain sees the unknown beyond beliefs and the conditioned laws of physics. You have to see it, be it, and live to be-live it. When our senses are finely tuned and synchronous, our perceptions are self-evident as truth. These experiences are beyond current science which denies the participatory nature of subjectivity experientially in daily life.

See the Significance of the Placebo Effect

In clinical trials, the effect of consciousness (and maybe time) is controlled for because it affects the outcome of the experiment. It's called the placebo effect. They measure the effect of a sugar pill or no treatment to subtract its effects from the overall effect of the experimental treatment. Often the treatment doesn't do much more than the placebo. The fact is human attention changes the outcome. The power of the placebo effect is often attributed to wishful thinking on the part of the study participant. Human attention is powerful. They also are receiving attention and maybe care by participating in the study. In mania, our brain is working fast enough so we can understand and insight how our subjective-participatory consciousness plays with life and the Universe in the moment. The same placebo effect scientific health studies control for is activated in human attention in mania. Human attention is magic. Human attention, care, and affection participates and effects the world. It changes what it beholds in untold and immeasurable ways. If we all had access to our magical attention, it would have a greater effect than any chemical treatment. We are all kept blind so we can be fed the products of double-blind studies. The drugs are to make up for our blindness! Our attention is our vision. The products are to compensate for our accumulated lack of attention. For example, when we ignore our health and make unhealthy choices, we may need a drug to compensate. When we walk in the world of magical attention, we don't need what we think we do in regular life. Living, flowing consciousness is the answer that rids many problems.

Momentary Marketing

Mania shows a greater source of energy than is typically available to human beings. It does a different kind of work. If we have little energy in a day, we might only watch TV. If we have a bit more energy, we go to work or become a success as it's currently defined. If we have even greater energy, we do something beyond the known jobs, actions, and successes of the world. It's up to us to declare our role to ourselves for ourselves. We aren't looking for the cause of mania but the source of it and its purpose.

The marketing of society tells us what life is about and what we should do. Mania is a state where the Universe markets the meaning of the moment to us. Mania course-corrects us towards what is meaningful to our core. Mania is 'expandicide.' We expand so much it destroys our ego, even if only temporarily. Expandicide has too many possibilities, even the possibility of going into disembodied dimensions. We are pulled in many directions. When possibilities die, it feels like death, and we can be in a state where we feel like we are dying, or we may as well die. Sometimes we can accidentally mistakenly destroy the body in confusion because we touch the boundary of where the body isn't designed to travel. Suicide can't see any other possibilities. Many who become enlightened die by expandicide, and they choose to leave the body. Maybe we don't attempt suicide but are tempted to leave by expandicide, which can appear as suicide in the Newtonian world.

How else can we look at expansion in mania? Let's take part of a quote by Don Estes shared in an earlier chapter. "Mind is the complex operator that resolves the difference between these opposites, and 'assembles' them together into manifested reality. The problems that arise in life do so to help resolve this tension." If we take the word mania and sprinkle it into Don Estes quote, we get "Mania is the complex operator that resolves the difference between [actual and potential self], and "assembles" them together into manifested {manic} reality. The problems that arise in life/{mania} do so to help resolve this tension." There is an ongoing tension between the false-self dying as we expand in possibilities in mania, and the possible-self dying after expanding as far as it can. The false-self re-engages at a lower energy state.

Morphogenetic Monkeys

J. Krishnamurti said, "Every human being is going through this hell, so if I as a human being understand this, I have discovered something which all human beings can discover."[98b] This extrapolates to one purpose of mania: to discover and harvest new information and make meaning out of it subjectively in the moment. In essence, he is saying when we discover something new, it makes it more discoverable by others. The discovery by one potentiates the discovery in the many, like the 100th Monkey Syndrome. It works through the morphogenetic field. We need to come closer together in consciousness to sync up. And the way we do that is by creating shared meaning and context. Because our gifts operate at a level more subtle than the everyday world, we don't need to connect physically or know what each other is doing. Just do the work that you do from where you do it, without attachment to the results. Results are in the realm of cause and effect, or Newtonianism. You can break the taboo of seeing and experiencing the positive side of bipolar. Eventually, as we integrate mania, we can make the positives chronic and persistent without the negative effects of getting carried away. Cultures with fewer years of experience with alcohol have a higher incidence of alcoholism because it takes time to adapt and learn to function with it as part of the culture. Though this isn't the best example, we can act manic to adapt to mania in the same way. Public intoxication is largely unacceptable, and so is public intoxication on mania.

Mania is co-consciousness with Gaia. That's why sometimes we feel like we are being punished when we don't act in accordance, or in a dance, with her. We can listen to the ego, or we can listen to Gaia. We are mediums of Gaia, and others can speak to Gaia through us. We are agents of magic. At the same time, as a humanity, we are all denying the magic element of ourselves. The magic is yet to flower. We don't have a context, space, container, or atmosphere for magic, so we manifest as manic relative to others who have no sense of magic. With no space for spontaneous magic play in society, normal people see us as fast-moving manics. It's a matter of relativity in consciousness.

If material reality vibed higher, we wouldn't seem manic relative to the predominant environment. It makes sense that regular-consciousness folks would perceive us as strange for finding life so exciting. From the mainstream energy level, life is accepted as mundane. Mania is based on different inner premises than mainstream reality, and because of this, we experience mania as if it has totally different physical premises. Premises is a good word to illustrate this because it can connote both physical place and inner values.

Bipolar is a punctuated, fluid, mutative form of growth into glimpses of enlightenment. The source is the truth of enlightenment. Unfortunately, we don't know much about enlightenment in the West, or what it's for. In mania, we usually use it for our own purposes and ends, so we can't stay in enlightenment. We are foolish and we fall back down to the minor leagues. If we look deeply, we can see the "source code," and we become the "sorcerer." The source code secret is inverting the source of words. Again, this doesn't mean that the brain-being won't shift back to the mainstream brain conformation after mania. We come back because our brains-beings-bodies are not designed to stay there. Someday, somenow, there will be no difference between the depths of our inner beings, our outer appearance, and the material world.

TRAUMA, TRANSFORMATION, SENSITIVITY, AND VIRTUAL REALITY

"Synchronicity is everywhere for those with the eyes to see it."

- Carl Jung

Sink or Sync

A mystic enters enlightenment without trauma, karma, or unfinished business. The same can't be said for the temporary enlightenment in mania. Mania partially disengages trauma to allow us to access the ecstasy beyond it. Even so, trauma pops up in mania and elevates to new heights in psychosis. In mania, we enter the realm of enlightenment with our trauma in tow. Since we have so much energy at our disposal, paradoxically, we can face some of our trauma during mania. We feel much stronger and can turn towards it and experience it. Mania is a natural trauma and karma-facing and healing mechanism. We can traverse something otherwise unbearable and bear to heal. Psychedelic-assisted therapy uses the same mechanism. Unfortunately, in mania we don't have someone to walk with us through the experience, bear witness, and keep us safe during our process. Bipolar people aren't told to pay attention to their experience for its own sake. We aren't told to ponder it and integrate it after. The intentionality of the experiences is what makes it about healing and growth. Even some newly designed psychedelic therapies can miss imbuing it with the intention to learn. Our culture doesn't educate us to be mindful of the possibility of having a crisis or spontaneous transformational experience at any point which we should pay extra intentional attention to. Imagine long before mania, being told about the possibility of a surge of energy, and that we are meant to learn from it. Imagine being told we'll have a deep dialogue about it after with elders who have gone through the process. If you haven't had mania, can you integrate this possibility into your psyche now? Can you tell others? Maybe mania only happens because of lack of attention to what matters in daily life. These missed moments add up to turn into a personal 4D movie that we must survive to come through the other side.

Energy and synchronicity put us a step or two ahead of our trauma. We can get so far ahead of ourselves that we get a glimpse of enlightenment. We can't stay there because of our trauma, so we are pulled back to Earth. This is our karma. We haven't taken all the steps required to get to enlightenment. Heck, some of us didn't even know about the concept of enlightenment, let alone the reality. Mania is an emergency bypass operation to disengage trauma that is dangerous to our existence. It buys us time. The Universe has a fight-or-flight mechanism too, and sometimes it propels certain beings into a higher state to sidestep an imminent danger. The trauma held in abeyance starts to release the longer we're awake in mania. We don't sleep enough to process our experiences through dreaming. What would be resolved in dreams has to be faced in daily life. And we can't sleep because we are facing our dreams and nightmares in waking material life. So, by being awake more in mania, we are given a chance to encounter in waking life what we usually sleep off in dreams. The world seems so dreamlike in mania because the dream resolution mechanism is active. We face dreamlike events in daily life. Our regular waking state isn't full wakefulness where we face life fully as we go.

Secret Sensitivities

Mania beholds secrets. My friend Katia pointed out that "it's a secret because people don't or can't understand." In mania, the secret is that we live fully now and thus are transformed. We can only be transformed by living fully in oneness now, not by living in abstractions. Yet we've been told to learn through abstractions. We are told to learn about life through concepts, then apply those concepts to life from memories. Living fully is only possible now, and then all is possible. Webster's dictionary defines transformation as, "The act of completely changing or altering in nature, form or function." Transformation is congruous with mania. We change completely in nature (Newtonian to quantum), form (from matter to frequency, energy, information, and light), and function (mediums of special messages, etc).

Sometimes I think of bipolar as Adult Onset Highly Sensitive Personhood (AOHSP) or Adult-Onset Empathetic Personality (AOEP). I might have been a highly sensitive child had I not decided to create a hard shell around me so that I didn't have to feel strong sensations. I remember when my heart hardened. One time I was walking to school with my little sister. She was five and I was seven. We were crossing at the busy intersection down the block when the metal clasp of her lunch kit gave way. The lonely apple inside fell out in slow motion, bounced on the pavement, and rolled to the bottom hill. After a perilous journey spinning uncontrollably down the steep hill, the dizzy, beat-up apple hit the curb, only to sit there defeated. A sinking feeling of sensitive panic overtook me. The poor little apple! I could sense the loving gesture of my mom putting the happy apple in the lunch kit. And now the apple was all alone. Not only that, but now my sister didn't have a snack for kindergarten. I felt sorry for the apple. I felt sorry for my sister. I felt sorry for my mom. After quickly working my sister up into a frazzle, we ran back home to get my sister another apple. I needed to confess the travesty of the apple's fate to my mom. I needed comfort. The whole drama felt painfully overwhelming. Even at that young age, I realized I couldn't go through life heartbroken over something like an apple. The gravity of my emotions gave way to numbing out my sensitivity as a survival mechanism. I gave up my highly sensitive personhood to protect myself from the pain and intensity of living. In my first mania, all the sensitivity I'd suppressed came rushing back. I found I wasn't adapted to operating with a full palate of sensations. I'd cut myself off from the opportunity to learn to live with sensitivity and grow my brain to adapt throughout my life. I had created a game of living with insensitivity, which I could handle and control. I didn't know how great the costs were going to be. In mania, some sensations felt raw and even painful.

Which World Witch Hunt

A person wearing a Virtual Reality headset acts strange because they react to the reality inside the headset, something the rest of us can't see. We wouldn't take a person experiencing another reality through VR to the doctor and ask for medication for an illness because we know they are experiencing an alternate reality mediated by the technology. Soon more and more people will have glasses with technology mediating alternate and augmented reality. People in mania are also experiencing an alternative reality mediated by the technology of the brain and the Universe. We are asked to medicate ours away. If we all knew how to augment our reality back to how it naturally should be, we'd be in a totally different world.

In some ways, mania is like spending too much time with a virtual reality headset on. Going into mania is like going into another reality without putting a headset on. We take off the consensus reality blinders. The longer we spend there, the longer it can take to reacclimatize back. The manic world is not the same thing as the consensus world. We take off the CR or "Consensus Reality" glasses and see with new eyes. When one person tries VR, they may tell others to try. Manic Reality is like VR but better. We can touch it, taste it, smell it, talk to it much more vividly. Everything seems meaningful and directly relevant to our life, as if handpicked by some futuristic AI algorithm. We do the fun things first—the synchronous things. One day, we'll lose track of whether we have a headset on or not. I've heard using a VR headset can sometimes make the user feel dizzy or sick afterward, and it can take a bit of time to re-equilibrate. It's the same after experiencing mania. Imagine if someone spent two months in a virtual reality world. What would happen once they removed the VR glasses? How would their brain be altered to make it difficult to function in regular life? Such a test obviously wouldn't be ethical. Hypothetically though, that person would be kept safe and cared for while they reacclimatized to consensus reality. They would need to relearn how to do things, just like we do.

Bandwidth High

In mania we get high on life because the now is full of energy. We get high on what is. What was is a downer. Mania is an attempt to associate with joy. We don't just disassociate from so-called reality but associate with another reality. Mania is solutionigenic— it generates a state of constructing meaning which is not passive but active and relies on subjective intelligence. When you see everything is one and in the now, you can decode any meaning by extrapolating from perception. Learning and teaching how to make meaning is imperative. The sooner we can do this, the sooner we can associate with Gaia now, rather than dissociating from the now into the past. We can inject meaning into the moment—faster than fearful interpretations from the past can interject. The past is always blind. Because it can't see the moment, what's happening now, the self as the past is innately afraid, whether it knows why or not. Far from bandwidth anxiety, manic people have bandwidth ecstasy and the joy of being embodied in eternity. Of course, no one talks about the bandwidth ecstasy because it's abnormal. Depression is normalized, while ecstasy is abnormal.

Mania challenges where information and energy come from. We think information and meaning come from outside of us. When we are generators of information and meaning, we can be beyond thought and the past through immediate perception-action. This is the source code of manifestation, and it's gestural. It leads to synchronicity, reality testing, and manifesting. It's a game-field where we get to figure things out from scratch instead of going off what everyone has told us. It's like starting over as a child, but as in an adult body. We need a new approach. In an email, Jamie Wheal of the Flow Genome Project said:

The disorienting experience of trying to map and plan for a future that's getting increasingly baffling, and it occurred to me that we're in need of what Thomas Kuhn famously called "a paradigm shift." His idea was that we have a model, or way of looking at things, and it mostly works. Except where it doesn't. Those error messages accumulate, until at some point, they force us to update or radically shift our model to reckon with all the error messages. Then we create a new more accurate paradigm until it also accumulates enough errors to force another upgrade.[99]

Mania is a paradigm shift. Special messages indicate errors in how we think reality is. In mania reality testing, we accumulate many error messages in how we are told reality works. We discover it doesn't work as advertised. We take a special interest in ourselves and capacities in mania to re-learn about ourselves. A child balances on one leg to see if they can. In mania, we do things to see if we can do them. Curiosity and reality testing are the keys that open the door to learn how reality really works. Our consciousness is participatory. Right now, we might accept that as theory. In mania, it's reality. It's a reality when we reclaim the energy that we are programed to waste by dividing and disconnecting ourselves from it. We feel a mission to create a paradigm shift so others can live it too. Quantum physics and Newtonian physics are different worlds.

EXPLORING POSSIBILITIES THROUGH METAPHORS OF MANIA

"Creativity is intelligence having fun."

- Albert Einstein

Not every insight into mania lends itself to a full paragraph. Here are some examples of short metaphors, similes, and analogies of mania. They are positive memes. They are subjective-pragmatic-participatory living experiencing informed lenses and perspectives. They are seeds for further flowering, unfolding, and exploration. Feel free to create your own memes of mania.

- Mania answers the question, what would you do with a ton of extra energy and time? What about extra curiosity, playfulness, and fearlessness?

- Mania relieves boredom and meaninglessness.

- Mania is a solution state.

- Mania does justice to being human.

- Mania is a resource that is untapped and allows us to tap our untapped resources, gifts, talents, and abilities.

- Mania answers the questions, "Is this all there is to life?"

- Mania is a state of information mining. Novel action in novel situation-spaces harvests information as perceptible through insight.

- Mania is a different choreographer of life.

- Mania is wild, untamed, and undomesticated.

- Mania is an involuntary state of overflow.

- In mania, we experience our star quality, magnetism, and charismatic nature.

- Mania is a burst towards self-actualization that sometimes neglects other basic needs on Maslow's hierarchy.

- Mania is innovative consciousness or innovation in consciousness. Mania is evolution innovating human consciousness.

- Mania is a super-trait with sub-traits within it.

- Mania is a learning style similar to our childhood learning style. We learn by experiencing and acting child-like.

- We are transported into a world where we taste our best potential self.

- In mania, everything feels urgent. There is an immediacy. There is no such thing as later, only now. This brings an intensity to the most mundane events.

- In mania, reality has a magical way of meeting our needs. When we need something, it's right there out of the blue, on the ground, or someone just happens to have it.

- In mania, we access other ways of knowing.

- Repetitive thoughts are dead words. Words in mania are alive, just like the space and everything in it. Words are given to us to say as living elements moving through us. Our language instinct is reactivated, and we can derive language from the moment and free associate memes.

- Mania is participatory and creative. We are temporarily outside the machine of society.

- Mania is a personal embodiment technology.

- Mania is a tangent reality or parallel reality.

- Mania is a micro-culture.

- Mania suspends the system of belief, or old meaning, so that we can perceive new meaning.

- In mania we go out and act "as if" the meaningful world exists because it does in a parallel reality.

- Mania is the victory state.

- In mania we dare to be happy for no reason. True happiness is beyond reason and logic. True happiness is always unreasonable. Reason won't take us to the new world. Only love of life will.

- Mania is a recreation state of the mind. Re-creation.

- In mania there is much more awareness and energy devoted to action, frolicking, wandering, shenanigans, laughter, play, reality testing etc., all of which do not require living according to the artificial clock.

- Mania is a luxury, so we live luxuriously.

- We never knew life could feel the way it feels until mania. And then we can't forget.

- Mood is related to possibilities. When our mood is ecstatic, there are ecstatic possibilities.

- Manics have different instincts and behaviors because we sense and process the world differently.

- Mania is magnetic, we attract ultra-original events.

- Mania creates the best possible scenarios and situations.

- Mania is a space to explore potential and see many possibilities.

- Mania is uncharted territory. The ego is the precedent we've set for ourselves, or that has been programmed into us. Mania is unprecedented. It's our unprecedented nature. It's our unpressed and un-dented being.

- We leverage the moment or now in mania. The rules of the system of the momentum of moments are pliable.

- Suddenly, certain aspects seem to be under our conscious control, and we can break the laws of physics like causality, time, space, gravity, energy, and matter.

- Mania attempts to write over old programming by living beyond it.

- Mania is learning to act without a formula. We don't know what to do. We can't rely on formulas living our life for us because they don't apply to aliveness.

- In mania the brain changes its structure to store less of the past, process more of the present, and build eternity.

- Mania is a new behavioral repertoire. Our suppressed originality breaks free.

- Mania is a rehearsal. We can try on the solution traits.

- Mania helps us discover our gifts. Remember your best manic traits and manic self.

- In mania, we adapt to a dynamic environment. The landscape is alive like a dreamscape.

- In mania, we are inquiring by acting, learning, adapting, and creating at the same time.

- Mania is an intrinsically motivated state, motivated by intrinsic energy.

- Mania is a fountain of youth.

- Mania is like making up for lost eternity.

- In mania, the Universe is questioning our human-created reality by showing us other possibilities. It's qualitatively and quantitatively different.

- In mania we fall in love with the Universe and Universe falls in love with us. The Universe is in love with our possibility, as our possibility is the possibility of the Universe.

- We're not excited to be manic. Existence is excited to be humanic—an ecstatic human being. Existence is looking for those who can embody the ecstasy.

- In mania, we try to find out if we are indeed eternal and immortal.

- Eventually, this feeling of amazement is no longer surprising to us or excitatory to the brain cells, and one can enjoy the fruits of the infinite kaleidoscope.

- The truth is alive. And it lives as you.

- When we no longer choose for ourselves from what we know, we feel chosen by the Universe.

- …

The words in this book could never come close to being a substitute for one second of mania yet the richness of mania could fill many volumes of words.

MANIC TRAITS AND SUPERPOWERS –
LIVING FASTER THAN A HEAD OF CONCEPTS

*"As it happens, Rickmansworth appears
on the first page of The Hitchhiker's Guide
to the Galaxy; it's the town where 'a girl
sitting on her own in a small café' suddenly
discovers the secret to making the world 'a
good and happy place.' But fate intervenes.
'Before she could get to a phone to
tell anyone about it, a terrible stupid
catastrophe occurred, and the idea was lost
forever."[d]*

- Shaun Raviv

Madly Adjusted

Psychiatrist Dr. David Cooper said, "Certain people have found a very discreet way of living out their madness. I think 'schizophrenics' tend to be victimized because they are not skilled enough in social tactics and strategy to do this in such a way that doesn't get them put away, locked up and tranquilized." He also said, "The symptoms of madness are the first sign of health," and "to suppress madness by drugs is to suppress the true self that needs to be developed."[56]

Rev. Martin Luther King coined the term "creative maladjustment." I think mania is a creative adjustment to a "mal" world, not that we are maladjusted. We step beyond the false world we've been programmed to, to be adjusted to, and see the actual world that is not based on illusory human concepts. There is a free world, and we must be free of the old world to access it. It's as close as our next perception and as far away as the whole collective human history.

During my first hospital stay, a relative of mine told me a psych ward psychologist said: "[One of the clinicians] said you went into some kind of dream world." I'm not sure if the psychologist meant metaphorically, that my mind went into its own world, or that there is a world that is dreamlike that I entered. It makes me wonder if they know what's going on at a higher level, or if sometimes the truth is communicated through clinicians too. There is a quantum world, and maybe they know that some people "go quantum" or go into some kind of dream world. The statement sounded exactly right to me. Maybe this whole book is a metaphor. Or maybe it's all a metaphor. The system is meant to keep the Newtonian paradigm alive. The old way wouldn't exist anymore if most people who'd ever gone crazy were supported through the stages of integration and shared their wisdom with the world. The problem is that the known world isn't willing to admit it doesn't know some things that 'crazy' people do, and to care to listen. It's easier to suppress it by calling it a problem of mental illness than admit that the world works in mysterious ways. Mental illness captures us, neutralizes the quantum rapture, and extinguishes integration.

The powers that be might know of the quantum possibility and train regular, well-meaning people to label it madness. At the same time, governments actively research and train people in remote viewing to gain intelligence into the defense operations of other countries. High-level government knows the capacity of remote viewing is real, and they harness it for their uses. They don't call it hallucination. The capacities are real, but unless the people in power can use them, they don't want us to learn to use them for ourselves and in egalitarian ways. Not only that, other powerful industries, like pharmaceuticals, make money by suppressing our powers—the powers of the people. The world isn't based on people accessing their gifts from the start of their life. Nor is it designed to help us find our lost gifts in adulthood. There'd be no need for fear, borders, or war if the people had their power because it'd be distributed. Out of fear, we look to authority for how we should be ruled. The majority of us are afraid, and fear is the main switch that turns our powers off.

Abilities Empowered

We can turn our powers back on just as easily. We acquire new abilities, skills, and traits overnight in mania, even if some of them are only temporary. We have new values, principles, and ethics that drive our needs, behaviors, actions, and mission. Something other than what was important is now important. We are powerful. These are some of the "manic/magic" traits that I feel I have access to because of the manic transformational crisis and metamorphosis:

> Energy, creativity, perception, spontaneity, possibility, outside the box thinking, meaning, reading between the lines, insight, ideation, generosity, kindness, innovation, manifestation, wonder, curiosity, re-languaging, neologisms, beauty, nature, magic, miracles, wholeness, oneness, integration, nonlinearity, spirituality,

questioning, dialogue, being childlike, comedic, silly, perceptive, insightful, sensitive, visionary, remote viewing, synchronicity, altruistic, best-self blueprint, playful, language creation, observant, presence, listener, creative, curious, trustworthy, open, intelligent, articulate, aware, prophecy, attentive, nature mysticism, understanding, resourceful, richness, quantum, lateral thinking, abstract thinking, etc.

With mania comes psycho-physical upgrades: Eyes, vision, sensation, voice, superhuman strength, hand-eye coordination, better balance, agility, posture, height, creative gestures, increased spontaneity, etc. We can also get what Mad Pride and Mind Freedom call "dangerous gifts." We humans are nowhere near finished with our development or evolution. We've been stunted and suppressed. We are behind, and that's why we can leap ahead in mania. A built-up pool of oppressed evolution should have happened by now, and when we get to critical mass, we are in store for a leap.

Mania enhances our abilities with no prior practice. They were there lying dormant the whole time, waiting for the veil to lift. But we can't maintain it indefinitely because the body takes longer to adapt through actions to being in that heightened energy than the operations of the mind. The body goes all out in the state of mania and spends all of its resources. Then the body needs rest in depression, or deep-rest. We sacrifice our time by going into depression, so it's important to harvest our mania to gather the fruits. We can pass on the wisdom to the kids. There is no reason why a child born today shouldn't be able to live out their dreams in material life. There need not be a gap. There are kids with multimillion dollar businesses. Wage slavery will be a thing of the past.

In mania, we access our "special powers" like premonition, prophecy, and other "siddhis." Most traditions warn against dabbling in them. When manic, I can "remote view." I'm not sure where I'm seeing, but I see people, things, and places with great clarity and detail. When it happens, I can feel my consciousness change its source, like putting my head in water and opening my eyes. What is your favorite superpower that you've discovered? I like changing the weather.

Shhhh!! Pass It On Through Peering

Once I met a man who had really big eyes. He told me a story of how someone passed on the gift to him, and he didn't always have eyes like that. He went on to explain we can pass on our gifts to people. His testimony confirmed my experiences where I'd had a similar insight. I realized we're meant to pass on our gifts to others holographically, through our eyes. This we can only do if we don't use our vision to pass judgments and projections. When we look with judgment, we add that projection to the energy pattern coming from our eyes, and people react or refuse to sustain eye contact. It changes the field of possibility for ourselves and others in the situation, and limits what waves functions can collapse. How the scenario plays out is trying to match what our brain is projecting. There is an invisible war of projected images going on between people. People trying to get 'what they want' or what they 'war.' This is what we're doing to each other.

If we could pass gifts and not judgments, this one simple thing would change the world in an instant. Imagine passing along positivity and possibility with our eyes. It's like passing on a download over airdrop. Even in a normal state, we can feel when someone is looking at us or perhaps has a bad intention. The energy in the room changes. We can pick up on energy, body language, and facial expression, which matches intention. Normally we can do this despite this capacity being atrophied by many orders of magnitude. In mania, we are more sensitive to all of this because we can take in and process more information. We might act on information that we don't even realize we are noticing. This is why sometimes other people are really surprised at how we are acting. We are picking up on how they are saying one thing, but their face and body are saying something else. We can't be fooled. In regular consciousness, we don't have the expansive energy or awareness to notice the incongruence like we do in mania. If everyone were manic, human beings would lose the capacity for deception because there'd be no point in trying. We are programmed to focus on words, on what people say, not the total field. We are programmed to waste our energy projecting lies, meanwhile, we can't sense the truth in another, and neither can they. It's a strange game. Imagine the thought experiment, 'what do we do when no one is looking?' Passing on judgments with our thought-projections is also 'what we do when no one is looking,' even though people are right there, within 'looking distance.' They can feel something. People in mania can feel that something ten times more intense. What is going on in your looking distance? You are re-patterning reality. Some of us can sense what people are thinking either by reading thoughts, reading face and body language, or by reading the situation and how it's playing out.

One day I was sitting in Tim Hortons, and I felt completely exhausted. Even though some time had passed since my last crisis, I was still regenerating. Every day I was tired, and the fatigue wouldn't leave me. Suddenly, my eyes met with a friendly stranger at the table across the way. He smiled and started speaking. He told me that he's a paramedic, though he was off work awaiting knee surgery. I told him I work in mental health. Though we only exchanged words for a minute or so, when we stopped talking and parted gazes, I realized that I no longer felt heavy or tired at all. It was a miracle from a friendly stranger. I knew again that energy can be passed through our eyes. We can be energized by good intention. Energy can have less to do with rest and sleep. There really is something about the light of a loving or friendly eye. We can be this for others and this could be how we magnetize strangers into higher states who give us special messages. It also speaks to the detrimental power of the clinical gaze. The quality of our gaze and what our eyes are silently saying are even more important now than ever, in a covered-up world. When we look from mania, we have a qualitatively different gaze. There is research that shows that in a manic state, pupils enlarge.[e] I think it has much to do with information and light coming in and out of our eyes, and how much energy we experience.

It's important to smile and make eye contact. It requires no physical contact. We make contact energetically, quantumly, holographically. We can hug each other through our gaze. Our body system can feel that yes, this is a friendly Universe. You can also "pass your genius" along or gift it to another through direct download through the eyes. It has been reported that bipolar people are sensitive to blue light.[f] I have a blue therapy light, and the box warns bipolar people not to use it. We can get too energized. Mania makes us sensitive to the information carried on light coming from the eyes of others. We can be so sensitive that we react to what others are projecting from their ego-eyes towards us. We can read their intentions.

Other times, we may get the feeling that we are invisible. We transform into our bio-electromagnetic light form. Many spiritual traditions say we have a subtle body made of light. I've experienced the light body many times. I call it our adjacent light body. It's a subtle, informational, spectral version of us that contains our possibilities since childhood. We are made of this light, and it emanates from our eyes. The spectral body can re-materialize the physical body. Rarely does the physical body act in alignment with our raw spectral data. It changes the posture, structure, and energetics of our physical body when it does. The energy of the nervous system moves freely, and there is more levity and less gravity. When we walk, we appear almost as if we are floating. Again, people tell me I look taller.

Many things that happen are too hard to describe in words. Only a small portion is retained in memory. Stories about what happened are less important than living it. Now that you know how much potential and possibility you have, what will you do with it? Is it possible to be consistently inconsistent and relentlessly ridiculous? We will get used to the synchronicity and coincidences. When we notice how plentiful synchronicity is, we can learn not to get too excited about it. We can discern which journeys to take and which invitations to decline. When we see the truth of abundance, we can choose our adventures and not go on everyone else's. Tangent realities can cause confusion until we see what synchronicities we wished for. Each time I experience mania, I strengthen the embodiment of who I really am and chip away more of who I'm not. The material world is like an elastic band that pulls us back. What happens when mania tips into psychosis?

Chapter 6

WHAT GOES UP MUST COME DOWN

THE TIPPING POINT - FROM MANIA INTO PSYCHOSIS

"Psychosis happens in the in between spaces of people, and the person who is psychotic bears the burden of making known this disruption in the in between spaces and so what you have to heal is the in between spaces and not the individual."

- *The Open Dialogue Approach*

The Flies on a Coconut

When I took training to become a rollerblading instructor, the first thing they taught us was how to fall, and how to teach people how to fall. Learning to fall safely is just as important as rising. We are bound to fall when we are learning of new ways and modes to move our bodies in space and time. As strange as it sounds, we can fall from mania better too.

Mania has shown me there are many possibilities out there and in here. Psychosis says game over, start again, you're at the end of exploring the many possibilities of mania, for now. It's like being a cat with nine lives or playing a video game with many lives. Psychosis is a re-start button. In some strange way, psychosis is a luxury. We get to start again from the beginning level of consciousness—fear fueled shame, guilt, and apathy. From there we can climb the stairway of consciousness, and experience new events at each level. Life gets progressively better.

The first time I experienced mania, I was flying high for a month with only two to four hours of sleep each night. When I couldn't fly any higher for any longer, I tipped over into psychosis. As mania was dying, I felt like I was too. It's scary to fall out of high states of consciousness, and fear is part of what helps to create the fall. Does fear make us fall or do we get afraid by falling? My first tipping point happened after an hour-long conversation with a dozen flies on a coconut. I was outside taking a photo of the mountain while drinking coconut water from a fresh coconut. After giving up on the photo and returning my attention to the coconut, I was surprised to find a fly chowing down on the top bit of coconut meat that remained after popping the top open with a meat cleaver. I started talking to the fly and he didn't seem to be afraid of me. At one point, he sat on the tip of my thumb, and he didn't move when I brought my nose within a couple inches. I turned my head away, and when I looked back again, he had invited his friends. There were half a dozen flies sitting on the coconut. Our conversation continued for about an hour. They sat there eating happily. They talked with me, though I did all the vocalizing. I could stick my finger a centimeter from their zillion eyes, and they remained unbothered. We started comparing flies and humans. A drama ensued and their actions showed that flies and humans aren't much different. The flies kicked each other, a big fly bullied a little fly, a fly went inside the coconut for more with near dire consequences, and then tried to fly off a ledge before he was dry. Sometimes they would fly straight at my forehead, bouncing off my third eye. In my meaning-making state, I interpreted that as them mistaking the light of my third eye as the light of the sun. They flew towards me instead of the sun. Had I become like the quality of light of the sun, and they couldn't tell the difference between my light and the sunlight? Was I as safe as the warmth of the sun?

Together, we co-created a story of how everything is interconnected, important, and has a role to play, including lowly flies. They were my friends, and they knew I wouldn't hurt them. It felt like I was in a heavenly world temporarily, where the "lion lays with the lamb," or the flies hang out with the soon-to-be-diagnosed crazy person. Time stood still and everything was one light. I made a video of the events on my iPhone 3GS (with no selfie camera), and when I watched it after, I was surprised by the drama that unfolded. I laughed uncontrollably as if I was watching the ridiculousness of someone else. After I stopped watching and laughing, suddenly everything felt heavy. The Universe felt like it was collapsing around me, like a scene in a movie where the camera zooms in rapidly and the music pitch warps as it lowers. I had reached a peak and tipped into the return. I felt pure terror as my mind was plagued with the full implications of my conversation with the flies.

The Terror-ible Truth

The Universe had unveiled its subtle secret truth of interconnection, oneness, and unity, and I'd just lived it. It wasn't a concept, it was embodied. I was it, the flies were it, the sun was it. The flies taught me many valuable lessons about life—that every part is valuable and sacred. At the same time, I realized that we humans don't really want to know this oneness, and that avoiding this fact is the source of all drama and violence. The drama is Maya, an illusion based on living out of touch with the truth of oneness. We don't already know this oneness beyond philosophy or concept because we can't face the truth. We can't face the truth, so we can't see it. We remain divided from it in our minds. The truth is intense, rich, beautiful, intelligent, alive and morphs quickly. Life grants us the wish to stay in the false darkness while talking conceptually about the light. It's our free will. Free will is categorically different from being free, which doesn't require will.

We must be in the light to be of, with, and as the light. There is a vast difference between talking "about" the light and speaking "as" the light. When we are the light, we speak as the light. We represent the light with our voice, not as the ego. This is the secret key mentioned before—to not preform the words you say is to speak as the light. Otherwise, our voice is the preformed dead sounds of the ego. Now I knew the truth, and I couldn't unknow—even if I wanted to. Not only did I know, now I could see the implications unfolding in each moment of each of my actions and the actions of others. The game of life changed to be more like a labyrinth of instant karma. I could see the error of my ways. I didn't know which way to turn. I felt like I was given dangerous knowledge. I could instantly see the dangers of acting in old paradigm ways, yet it was hard to act in right, light, new paradigm ways in a dark world. I didn't know if I could make up for my mistakes at the same time. I couldn't forgive myself. I was in limbo, unfit for either world.

As the heavy darkness clouded out the light, I wanted to run from the darkness and my part in it. I ran from the dark and chased myself into the dark knight of the soul. Run! We are all actually connected—ONE!! How can it be dangerous to know the truth? The old paradigm world of Maya would not hold up in the light of the truth. The game of truth is the ultimate challenge in embodiment. Being and living as one in oneness is an ultra-marathon from awakening to the tipping point back. I had been there for a month, and now the darkness of separation was returning. The return of darkness is a life-and-death situation. I didn't know how long I could last with the awareness of oneness and the weight of my karma. I was in crisis. My memories were mixing with the moment, creating terrifying experiences. If everybody realized oneness instantly, mass hysteria would ensue. We'd go crazy in the plume of the residue of what we did when we knew not what we were doing. And we'd go crazy trying to do the right thing now and now and now, in a world designed out of sync with oneness.

The realizations continued. This is everybody's fault! And so it's nobody's fault! And it's all my fault!! I did this!!! When all is one, there's no blame or cause. We are addicted to causality, and we only know how to act out of our addiction. We're addicted to seeing division with our thoughts—better, worse, good, bad, blame, shame, ugly. Thought chatter is second-guessing oneness and being out of sync with it. It's not trusting the truth of the moment. All thoughts are second-guessing what the moment would otherwise inform us. And it's always been this way, so there's nothing to do. The Universe is a genius! We're all in it. We're all doing it. And we can't see it. We can't see the truth. And I just saw it! And now I can't unsee it!! I can't see it anymore, but I know it!! I know too much! And I can feel it! I can feel too much! Am I going crazy? I'm going CRAZY! I'm CRAZY!!

The Trick is the Past

I ran to try to escape from the self, only to end up like the guy at the end of the Radiohead music video for the song "Just"– lying down, unable to move. Running from the self is fear and fear is the self. Running, turning away, is the self. The self and its chatter, thinking it knows better, warps, and distorts us from the light. The ego has a refractory index, just like water and other materials that light can pass through. In mania, fear disengages. Now it's reengaged. The false-self escapes from the moment and that maintains the false-self. I couldn't turn the other cheek. I couldn't face myself and the karma of my life, my previous lives, my possible parallel lives, my family constellation, the whole of human existence, and the cosmos. That karma seeped into the light dimension and extreme ecstasy tipped into extreme terror.

I usually tip from mania to psychosis when I get the feeling "I know too much." It started with, "she knows too much," and I thought people were coming to take my bipolar notebooks full of insights. It morphed into "I know too much." In later iterations of psychosis, I experienced feeling like a homeless man. When this happens, I know my brain took one inevitable step too far, like a cow unknowingly trying to go outside an invisible electric fence. I inadvertently stepped beyond the unknown invisible energetic barrier, and there's a psycho-physical shock. I "turn back" running, just like the cow. I know I've gone as far as I can this time. Possibility recoils, inverts, and folds back up. I went beyond the impossible, and I know too much. The brain can't handle infinity and immortality. To stay a human being, we must turn back.

The physiological response is swift. The terror is impossible to quell. Fight or flight kicks in. As soon as we start running or retreating, we feel like something is after us. Eventually we may need to wave the white flag and surrender to the psych ward. This is when I freeze in terror. Once we retreat, we likely need treatment. After the transition, it's hard to calm the nervous system on our own. Then we go to the psych ward, making it a nightmare. The medications can help. A good tranquiller can help us wake up in the sleepwalking world. Now we're in a bad dream. Psychiatry calls it psychosis.

The Burn of the Return

We haven't reached critical mass for the new paradigm, so going back is a necessary evil. We can't go too far into the new way of being without, at some point, becoming unreachable and un-relatable to our old-world friends. If we continue, eventually we'll be dealing with more energy than the body is designed to handle on its own. We need other people with us to spread out the energy. If we don't have more people, we have to go back. It's the same as going scuba diving with at least one other person because it's dangerous to go alone. Getting terrorized into turning back is part of the grand design so that we can participate in a paradigm shift in humanity. Otherwise, we'd all stay there and leave others behind. Some choose not to go back, hence the high "suicide" rate appearing in the world of Maya. One day we will sync up in our iterations like fireflies and gain momentum for returning power to the people.

Perhaps one day, instead of running away, we won't feel afraid of psychosis at all. Maybe psychosis is made worse by the fear of the fear in psychosis. Rupert Spira has a great YouTube video called "Why are you so afraid of the fear."[100] He talks about *being* with fear rather than getting rid of it and that we have to learn to live with fear before we can live without fear. This takes courage. I found his video helpful for gaining perspective on the fear of fear in psychosis. This is highly relevant since we are told implicitly or explicitly when we get diagnosed to be afraid of ourselves. A diagnosis implies that we mistrust ourselves, so any sign or "symptom" generates fear rather than curiosity or learning. We think the professionals know better. And perhaps they do at first, but fear can prevent us from trying to learn for ourselves. We default to thinking we are experiencing a symptom we should be afraid of, and act to stop it immediately. Cortisol, which is released when we are stressed, prevents learning and thinking straight. Part of psychosis is not being able to think straight, so we make it worse by being afraid of it. We're afraid because we don't know how to be with fearful content, without fear.

Fear Street

It's important to address the fear of fear. If we can transform the fear of fear, and behold what's happening without fear, it transforms the fearful content into something else. Maybe the "symptom" or the fear is something else, but it can't reveal itself or communicate anything when we are afraid of it. We can use our placebo powers when we rid ourselves of the fear of fear, because the light of our attention without fear has a transmutative and alchemical power. Just like when we gaze at another without judgment, it works when we gaze at our 'symptoms' too, without fear. Fear is a judgement. We've been told to look at symptoms psychiatrically, which is imbued with fear. It works whether we are looking inside or outside. We can stop the fear from snowballing. Taking a class like the Wellness Recovery Action Plan plants the seeds of self-empowerment to address triggers, warning signs, and more in a personal plan. The WRAP app is a free download.

Once when I was in a major crisis, I used the technique that Rupert Spira describes in his video. He starts with "Why are you afraid of the fear?" I experienced feeling a potent substance releasing in my heart, like black ink from an octopus. The substance felt like it was an infection of pure terror and evil. My heart was pounding, and I had a strong thought to call 9-1-1. I could see how the fear was trying to control me, like a subtle holographic pattern. The black ink diffused and quickly permeated my entire body. Though I'd experienced psychosis five times by that point, I'd never experienced my heart leaking evil ink before. Psychosis is a trickster, always changing the game. The trickster wanted to trick me into being afraid of that fearful sensation. It wanted me to call for help, for me to go the psych ward, and turn into a mental patient.

I listened to Rupert Spira's video, and it supported me to not be afraid of the fear. I thought I would need to get help, but I didn't thanks to following his words. The false-self is the entity that is afraid. After several minutes the fear and physical pain subsided. I maintained a state of not being afraid of the fear. I avoided creating that other layer of fear. The fear was there, the pain was there, but there was no fear of it. I didn't try to do anything about it, just be with it and give it attention. I didn't separate myself from it by identifying as the person who doesn't accept fear. When I identify with something, I take myself to be something separate. Because of that, I was free to go through the fear with acceptance and surrender. I knew I could handle it because I wasn't adding to it. I didn't act out of fear, so fight or flight didn't kick in. Initially, I had to freeze, then I was able to align with the process and not resist it. After freezing, I was in a free state, and I was free to be one with the fear. At the same time, I was ready to call for help if I needed it. That time, I never did. I was able to get through a full-blown crisis by myself at a peaceful retreat rather than a chaotic, re-traumatizing psych ward. I learned that I could become stronger and face psychosis and be present with some of it. The more I learn to do this, the less chance I'll need escalating amounts of medications over time that will impact my health and functionality in negative ways. It's not true that each episode creates worsening of the condition over time if we care to learn about ourselves. There was a time years later where I intentionally let a mania get out of hand and I did have to go to the hospital. I drove myself there.

Thoughts create a labyrinth that challenge us to get back to the mainstream world. Many pitfalls feel like death traps. The psych system is a trap that is a step above the death trap, trying to save us from death while at the same time seeming like they are trying to cause it. Since we were expecting death, being trapped in the psych system can feel hopeless. But they are trying to keep us alive. It's a pseudo-human created mercy where we wait for mercy. It's where we can wait out our fear of the death traps instead of remaining vulnerable wandering in the dark of society. We can feel attacked by thoughts, the past, entities, sensations, karma, people, or quantum weirdness that comes to mess with our beliefs about reality and ourselves. Sometimes it feels cruel, like a test, punishment, or torture. We run through the labyrinth until we collapse with fingers crossed, praying for mercy. The psych ward is a place to go through these lower levels. I don't think it causes it.

THE STRANGE VALUE OF AWE IN THE SCENARIOS, TIMELINES, AND PARALLEL WORLDS OF PSYCHOSIS

"The mind, Ray, can sometimes create and alternate reality, a false reality, to shield itself from trauma. From the things we fear, from the horrors we can't even imagine."

- Fractured, the Movie

At Esalen in the summer of 1968, there was a conference called "The Value of Psychotic Experience." Presenters included Alan Watts, Stan Groff, R.D. Laing, John Weir Perry, and Allen Ginsberg. Seeing that there is value in psychosis is nothing new. Bipolar, mania, and psychosis are part of the human experience and thus part of human nature. According to futurist Jason Silva, "Awe is an experience of such perceptual vastness you literally have to reconfigure your mental models of the world to assimilate it."[101] Mania and psychosis are part of awe because our mental models have to expand to assimilate them. As our experience expands in mania, awe ensues because our mental models try to inflate to make sense of it. Mania is supra-awe, or beyond awe, in that it quickly and profoundly reconfigures our mental models for us. We don't have to try to get the software download and start the install. The process of ego re-engagement is like awe-reversal or reversing the awe. The inertia of awe and synchronicity went on for a prolonged period and now the field of ego consciousness re-envelops the body-mind. New meaning and metaphors that enchanted us in mania are replaced by the haunting old nightmarish illusions of psychosis. They have an inertial force equal and opposite mania to pull us back.

Psychosis feels like the Universe is running scenarios. The theory of the Multiverse says that all possibilities that ever could exist do so now; a new Universe is created from every decision point and so they are theoretically accessible. The algorithm of the Universe unfolds possibilities as scenarios as it doesn't have the computational capacity to unfold all Universes at once, or at least the human brain doesn't. Human participatory perception decides what to render and create. Just as some people have multiple personalities, the experience of psychosis feels like having "multiple scenarios," or multiple worlds running at once, and we can access different scenarios based on different decisions at different moments. We may be able to jump from one decision timeline to another and back again. Our world is no longer based on linear time but attending to different worlds of different levels of consciousness. Each person we meet creates a new world because of their level of consciousness too. Since all possibilities exist now, it seems likely that a few possibilities could render themselves simultaneously in one individual consciousness if our mental models reconfigured to allow it.

Maybe this is a way for some of us to choose a better scenario, or destiny, rather than be fated by the limited scenarios of the false-self algorithm. Preventing our trans-conscious missions with a permanent mental illness label may be detrimental to the evolution of consciousness. We are supposed to be finding our destiny. Since we don't know how to enter synchronicity to do so, we are fated to be mental patients. But the Universe is patient, and it's waiting for us to choose again. Each iteration of mania and psychosis trains us how to play the game of selecting scenarios or destiny better. That is, if we decide to learn from it each time rather than be afraid. The process is out of the field of time, so it doesn't matter if we get it right in the linear world. It matters that each time, we gather the puzzle pieces while we are in a heightened state and consciously integrate them after. Our character changes depending on what we select.

A talk by Deloris Cannon goes into the idea of the "background people," that not all people are really real, but are appearances. In a YouTube video titled "We Are All Living Parallel Lives" she said this to answer a question about schizophrenia:

> Some of these people are more aware and awake than we give them credit for. Too many people are channeling now. The definition for schizophrenia was channeling—they are seeing all the options and split offs, they see all the other lives, they can see other dimensions. In some instances, some individuals

are actually connected with other aspects of themselves that are in different lives, in different parts of the world and different parts of the Universe and they are experiencing it concurrently, and people living in a single way don't understand it so we institutionalize them because we don't understand it. The veil is so thin.[102]

More people need to know this. Parallel worlds imply stepping into the "adjacent possible," as Jason Silva puts it.[103] Multiple possibilities are happening at once. Understanding there are multiple parallel worlds, it's easy to see how we might see more than one reality at once. We can see something that's in another reality. It's called a hallucination or seeing something that isn't there, but it's there for those who can see more than one reality. Hallucinations are artifacts of another reality, or of the holographic nature of the Universe. If we take what the frontiers of physics say about simulation, holographic, and quantum theory, none of our experiences are weird or hallucinations, but we are living examples of their theories, that are reality.

Why don't we get to sit with those scientists and tell them our experiences to confirm their theories, rather than sitting with psychiatrists to spill our 'symptoms.' We are waiting for a paradigm shift. It remains locked in theories of science and away from who it's happening to in everyday life. The theories are real in everyday life, but everything is reversed. What is visible to someone with schizophrenia holographically, when corroborated by others that can see, it will be visible to non-experiencers. We won't be able to confirm it if we are isolated from each other thinking about our illness. We can go into a parallel reality and come back. It's not that weird. We just need to get used to it to the point where we talk about it in a relaxed manner. Like sharing what we had for dinner. It's no big deal. It's made to be a big deal because there is no profit when we are all prophets. Beau Lotto said human beings are "adapted to adapt."[104] The thought that we can't adapt to quantum weirdness is maladaptive. In the state of mania, our brain makes salient the information and perception of parallel realties, possible futures, and the possibilities mentioned by Deloris Cannon about schizophrenia.

A STORY OF DEATH AND REBIRTH – COLLAPSING ROGUE WAVE FUNCTIONS TO RESOLVE OVERLAPPING IMPOSSIBILITIES

"The secret to life is to die before you die –
and realize there is no death."

- Eckhart Tolle.

What is it like to peak in mania only to stumble into psychosis? I call it hitting the wall. I read in the book *The Celestine Vision* that "'the wall' is that feeling we can go no further."[105] For me it feels like I've gone too far and know too much.

The first time I had a month-long psychosis after a month-long mania, I re-experienced my birth. Not only that, but I also simultaneously experienced giving birth to myself. I was breathing in and out in a rhythm that I later learned is used in "Holotropic Breathwork." Right before I started breathing rhythmically, I felt as if I was dying, for real. I panicked and wanted to jump in a cab and take a train to California, but I knew the day before was my last chance to escape. Now I didn't have the strength. I went to another room to ask my friend if she could help me "fake my own death." She shook her head no and rolled over to go back to sleep. I viscerally felt like I was running out of time as if there was a physical and metaphorical clock ticking down. My body was that clock, and it was running out of time. I could feel the weight of the world crushing me as the pull of gravity got stronger and stronger. My heart was racing, and I was pacing around, realizing there was no possibility of escape. I felt like something was after me and going to kill me any second or that I might harm someone out of confusion. I was absolutely terrified. I felt like I was trapped in the World Trade Center with the choice to burn alive or jump to my death, a no-win situation. I panicked and I felt the urge to run and jump off the second-floor balcony. I felt like soon I'd fall over, and I wouldn't be able to get up because I was too weak, and gravity was too strong. I felt like my bowels were going to evacuate and, to put it nicely, extreme sexual energy in my root chakra. I peed on a pee pad on the floor that I had from a medical test. My hair had been falling out in heaps, and I weighed only 90 pounds.

In a flash, I knew how I could stop myself and save my own life. When I was eight years old, I purchased a pair of handcuffs from a yard sale at a house at the bottom of the lane for $1.80 in dimes. Luckily, I remembered where I'd put them, so I bolted across the room and grabbed them from the right-side, bottom closet drawer. I ran to the balcony and attached one cuff to the lower horizontal railing and the other cuff to my wrist. Instead of jumping off the balcony, I jumped into a sleeping bag I had left on the balcony from the night before when a similar process was happening. I wanted to sleep under the open sky where the Universe could see and save me from the things that only happen behind closed doors. I was physically safe, and others were safe from me. I could surrender to the process that I couldn't escape. I was fine with lying there, helpless, with the possibility of being harmed as long as I couldn't harm anyone else. I felt overwhelming terror that vampires were going to kill me, while at the same time it was better than harming someone and then jumping off the balcony. The terror was intense and now I had no choice but to be with it and go through it.

To start, I had a vision of seeing my friend after she bit me like a vampire and there was blood all over her face. As I lay there facing south towards Mount Baker, I decided to keep my eyes shut. Before I handcuffed myself, I "tried to kill myself" with a gesture of eating a lot of honey and yacon syrup, which is like fancy molasses. Something told me that doing so would put me in an insulin coma, the process would stop, and I'd wake up in a hospital and not remember anything. Coincidently the system put mental patients into comas by injecting them with insulin.[106] I felt like I might wake up in a parallel world and they'd tell me I fell while rollerblading in California and hit my head, rather than becoming a mental patient. The yacon syrup got on my arm and, at one point, when I did briefly open my eyes, I saw what looked like blood.

I'd collapsed and experienced several possibilities of dying or being in a coma, and that's when I began to give birth to myself. I was breathing forcefully in and out. The breathing happened on its own. It felt like something was expanding and collapsing my rib cage and diaphragm, like a fire blower. At the same time, I felt like I was in the birth canal. By giving birth to myself, I was remembering my birth. I can remember that I experienced every aspect of my birth intensely at the time, though now I can only remember the subtle knowledge of re-experiencing all of it. I had to give birth to myself because I had just died or was near death. After giving birth to myself, I had several powerful experiences. They felt like they were happening in a realm of limbo where many energies and possibilities were trying to resolve themselves. It felt like I had rebirthed myself, but there was still no guarantee I'd make it through alive again. I had no idea what was going to happen or what was happening. I just had to surrender and let it happen—especially because I had given myself no choice being handcuffed.

At one point in the night, I felt I was a bird in a flock flying south. I felt the subjectivity and experience of the bird flying in formation—the rapid heartbeat, the flapping wings, and I could hear myself and other birds tweeting. One side of my mouth was opening and quivering with each tweet. I was hoping I was flying south and would land in Santa Barbara. If I couldn't take the train, I'd fly as a bird. Something told me I'd wake up as a homeless man that had been sleeping on the beach and my whole life would've been just one of his nighttime dreams. Yet, at the same time, I would have lived physically and had indeed died—so many paradoxes. I also experienced being a homeless man, but I was lying on State Street, with my eyes closed. I could hear the bustle and talk of everyone walking by as I lay there unnoticed. Later, I experienced an angelic being trying to lift me from my body. I felt the warmth of her presence, and I could see the white light. As I felt her lift me up, I felt a sense of joy and I could feel my facial muscles form a huge smile. Then my arm stretched to a halt by the self-imposed handcuff. I could feel the pain of the unforgiving metal on my wrist. By handcuffing myself, I had made a gesture of wanting to stay on Earth and ensured my stay.

At some point in the morning, my friend came into the room, and I tried to convince her to help me fake my death again. She refused, citing she had to go to work. Later I heard someone say my name with a questioning inflection. And then I heard, "Call 9-1-1." I felt someone flipping me from my side onto my back towards them. As I rolled over, I felt myself file through several other possible endings to my life. One that I recall is that I was at the scene of a car accident or lying outside of a car on the ground all bloodied up. I experienced my family rushing to come to see me there, barely alive, saying my name to try to wake me up. Were these the deaths I escaped in tangent worlds or possible future deaths? Being flipped over collapsed the quantum wave function around me. In my mind, I was at the scene of a car accident. I heard my younger brother say my name. I couldn't and didn't open my eyes. I thought I was dead and so did they. Perhaps I was catatonic. The paramedic showed up and I didn't respond, thinking I was dead. It wasn't until the medic squeezed my finger joint to see if I was conscious that I knew I was alive. It hurt and I winced. I don't remember seeing anyone—my family, the medic, my room. I don't have any memory of opening my eyes. I was told I walked to the ambulance on my own, though I have no memory of walking or having my eyes open. I vaguely remember being in the ambulance on the way to the hospital. The ride was bumpy and dark. They didn't let any family come with me, which was strange. All I experienced was darkness, and it felt like I was in a hearse. I have no recollection of the inside of the ambulance. The first time I saw anything was when I opened my eyes in the hospital. I was lying on a gurney. I stared at the clock for what seemed like more than a couple of minutes and the time didn't change. I felt like I could dilate time.

All of this occurred over eight to ten hours. It felt like I was hopping realities to get back into synch with mainstream time because I'd gone too far. I had managed to come back to life in this world after going far off into consciousness. It felt like I died in a parallel world, and I experienced the struggle to bring myself back to life on a similar but different timeline. A timeline where I hadn't died and everyone I loved was in the same world. There was a possibility where I was killed, but I escaped it. I had to come back. My death was then just a nightmare. If you want to see a depiction of this, watch the first episode of *The OA*.

After experiencing many vast shifts in consciousness, including mania and terrifying psychoses, I feel trained up for today's times. Psychosis now feels like an asset as I understand how to keep myself safe and not panic in a crisis—I'm a paramanic. I can endure a crushing amount of psycho-somatic pain. I can resist the reflex to act panicked if panic ensues.

HITTING THE WALL – DISSOCIATION, CRISIS, CAPTURE, AND OUTSMARTING SUICIDE

"Given the illusion of objectivity, a psychiatric diagnosis should be a description rather than pretending to depict an immutable reality that is observable by everyone in all contexts."

- *Mel Schwartz*

After my experience of death and rebirth, that strange ambulance ride to the hospital, then lying there on the gurney, I found myself sitting up at the end of a bed in the triage area. A nurse started interrogating me. As she hunched over me, she yelled "What's going on?" I had no voice, but I wanted to tell her the sad truth that I felt in my heart. "We are killing each other with our thoughts, feelings, and actions." I could feel the gravity, texture, weight, depth, pain, and sorrow of those words with every cell of my body. I could hear the words in my mind's ear, but I couldn't say them. I knew she wouldn't get it, so what was the point? She didn't want to get it.

Though I had just been on an epic deep inner-space journey, then soared to cosmic heights, ending in facing death, I felt so dejected, hopeless, and crushed from the realization I had fallen from grace back into the Matrix. I couldn't stay in the new world, and I was sent back to the past world. I had travelled to the future, which is just the present moment relative to living in the past. There wouldn't be any illusory Maya reality to come back to, only the truth of oneness in the eternal present if we all saw this. In mania, I was sharing my insights with everyone who I encountered. I once heard this referred to in clinical terms, as "wooing strangers." Funny, it doesn't sound very technical. Now I knew there was no point in speaking to deaf ears, blind eyes, closed hands, and grey hearts.

The nurse quickly grew impatient with her despondent patient. My silence made her lift her head and yell "security." In response, I quickly scooted my 90-pound butt off the triage bed and ran through the hospital's sliding doors in my socks. I dashed across the road, hurdling through thirty feet of thick brush, and sat down in a muddy patch among tree roots on the riverbank. I played with clay, listening to the salient sound of hovering helicopters, convinced they were looking for me. My clothes were soaked with mud and my body started shivering uncontrollably. I knew I had to choose between the cold or the helicopters getting me. I wandered up from the riverbank and happened upon a couple who were out for a stroll. They let me use their cellphone. I wanted to call a friend, but I didn't know anyone's number. Those strangers were more compassionate than the nurse at the hospital and offered to drive me home. Though I was coated in mud, they wrapped me in a blanket and helped me into the back seat. On the short drive back, they said their daughter was an ER nurse at the hospital I'd just fled. Psychosis is dotted with irony and dark synchronicity. I must have rolled all three of my eyes.

When I got home, my younger brother was there to greet me at the street and ushered me to his house next door. Everything looked holographic, including my brother. After showering, my sister came into the bathroom to tell me the police were there to take me to the hospital. I was cornered and trapped. I agreed to go in peace, as long as she could go with me. The police said they had to put me in handcuffs—more irony since I'd just handcuffed myself. Back at the hospital, I was sitting beside my sister. My brother sat across from us, and the police officer stood next to him. None of them looked at me or said anything to me the whole time. The heaviness started again, and I found myself on the floor, holding onto my sister's leg while sliding down it. We waited hours before the psych intake nurse poked her head out to call me into the room. She opened the door the moment I thought I couldn't take the crushing sensation another second.

Mercy. I distinctly recall a smirk on my brother's holographic face as I was handed over. Strange imposter. The nurse asked me a bunch of questions, each time, lowering her voice, chin, pace of speech, while looking over her glasses as if to induce me to tell the truth. The accuracy of her questions made me wonder how she knew what I was experiencing. How did she know I could read people's thoughts? She must be able to read mine. I answered truthfully to all the questions but one—whether I was getting special messages from the TV. I was, and I knew I'd receive extra punishment if I admitted that. I spent three days in an isolation room waiting to get a bed in the psych ward. I felt so safe and relieved in the small square room. All the sources of information overload were cut off, and I was tranquilized. No one could get me. I'd sit up and peek out the door to see a nurse behind a high counter look back at me. She smiled, and I felt so reassured. My safe feeling ended when I got up to the psych ward.

I've been to the psych ward six times each time, getting there became easier. The first time, I went in handcuffs. I had to go back for a second stay four weeks after the first because I developed flat affect and severe akathisia from the medication they put me on. A family member drove me in that time. The third time, I went in an ambulance because I was too terrified to get in the back of the car. The fourth time, my peer support supervisor drove me. The fifth time, a friend who works in the system drove me and got me in quick. The sixth, seventh, and eighth times, I got through it without going to the psych ward. I learned to navigate crises on my own because, on my fourth visit, the psych ward doctor traumatized me. She put me on similar medications to very first time I was hospitalized, even though I asked her not to because of my history with a terrible reaction. The ninth time,

I drove myself to the mental health center for an intake, and a clinician took me to the hospital so I could get in faster. I had let things go too long and get out of hand. I needed professional help. It's gotten easier and less dramatic over time.

Besides the one traumatic psych ward stay, overall, I've had positive experiences and been treated well. In these vulnerable states, we need care and compassion. I have hope that one day compassion will form the foundation of a transformation-friendly mental health system, as shared by Ron Unger. Until then, it's helpful to freeze in crisis rather than fight or flee. It's mercy and compassion for others to not create drama with fight or flight. Others don't understand what we are going through. When you feel like you can go no further, call for help, take the treatment, and rest. Waking up in the psych ward can feel meaningless and hopeless, but it can also feel like time travel. We think we can go no further, but we can. Mercy is real. Rest, binge-watch Netflix, sleep 14 hours a night. Whatever you need to do. Live as fully as possible when you can.

MORE STRANGE CRISIS EXPERIENCES AND EERILY ACCURATE CINEMATIC DEPICTIONS OF MANIA AND PSYCHOSIS

"The psyche of a small minority of individuals, in comparison with that of the overwhelming mass, is constituted by both greater depths and a higher degrees of turmoil. To ensure they're not torn asunder by the conflicts, contradictions and abysses within, such individuals are driven to explore and impose order on their psyche, fashioning and sculpting themselves into a harmonious totality."

- Friedrich Nietzsche

When Enough is Enough for Now

In crisis, believing that it's all just my mental illness sometimes comes as a welcome relief. I've seen many glitches in the Matrix! I've also had a stigmata-like experience when I was in a crisis state. I went to psych emergency, and they turned me away, likely because they were too full, so I went home with an additional prescription. When I got home, I walked in the door only to see blood on a red pepper sitting on the counter. I dabbed it with my finger and tasted it because I was sure it wasn't blood. I tasted blood. A family member was there, I started interrogating them, asking them and the Universe "what's going on?"—a bit like the triage nurse years earlier. I remember their behavior became nonsensical, backing up hysterical, almost as if I were physically attacking them. I can still see it distinctly in my mind's eye. In retrospect, some of these scenarios felt like family constellation therapy, but played out with my family. Were we playing out violent scenes of the past? Were they clues to what's happened sometime in my family lineage? That stuff doesn't leave the DNA. Perhaps we had shared psychosis where they were drawn into it. I have no idea what happened after that. I do have a picture of the bloody red pepper somewhere. At the time I had a bunch of coconuts in the fridge, and I couldn't open the door because I thought I would find heads inside. I had an intense feeling of merging the energy of a murderous pedophile, though I experienced the possibility of these actions as horrifying. I felt like maybe it was a past life reincarnation and I was feeling the karma of what I'd done then. Sometimes I have a sense of past, parallel, or future lives that range from devastatingly evil to omnisciently ecstatic; from one end of the spectrum of possibilities of being human to the other. In a sense, I've lived all possible lives, the sense of which is immense and frightening. I am that, I am all, and that leaves no place for judgment. Can I divide myself from another and pretend they're not me too? It's all part of the human psyche that we share and stare at each other from ever exchanging bare bodies. The "me" divided from "you" and all the games that arise from the use of these two pronouns while using them to divide the one life that cannot be divided. This whole equation of language is false and unfounded mathematics. I ended up in a different psych ward a couple of days later.

Waking Up Walking in Where Am I?

One time I was learning how to take a particular regime of vitamins, minerals, supplements, and remedies to take less medication. What I took varied depending on how I was feeling. At the time, my bipolar biorhythm was a cycle of six months of wellness, crisis, and then three months of recovery. I was taking the supplements for some months when I had a strange experience while trying to fall asleep. As part of the protocol, I was sleeping in a totally dark room for maximal melatonin production in my brain. I was lying there as usual, and when I turned over, suddenly, I felt this vast emptiness. It was as if I was being lifted until I was out in the cosmos. I could feel my body breathing gently as though it was breathing by itself. There was an immense feeling of peace. Even though I was wide awake with my eyes closed, I felt like I had my eyes open inside, looking inside at the darkness, and my body felt like it was still. At some point I felt like I'd gone too far, and I couldn't stay like that forever, and I wanted to end the experience. With effort, I pulled my consciousness back to my body. I got up from bed and took more vitamins to fall asleep for real, as per the protocol. I remember going back to bed and then soon getting up to take even more vitamins.

This time, right when I got back into bed, instantly I realized that I was sleeping, without any time to fall asleep. It felt like I'd been asleep the whole time. At the same time, I was still wide awake and got up right away, but it was like getting up from a dream after sleeping. I started to get desperate, not knowing if I'd been awake or dreaming. It was like I was in the movie *Inception*, though I didn't think about that at the time. I took more vitamins and tried to sleep on the couch. By this point it was around 4:00am and I still couldn't sleep. I was a bit scared, and I didn't want to take more medication because I was trying so hard to minimize it. I went back to bed to try one more time to fall asleep. As I lay there trying to fall asleep, and not knowing which reality I was in, out of nowhere, I heard a mystical voice say, "you've taken too many supplements and you need to medicate yourself." I don't hear voices, not even my own voice, but that one was loud and clear. I took some medication, and a bit more, and more until I fell asleep. Sometimes hitting the wall is not being able to sleep. The voice taught me that there comes a time for some extra medication, no matter how determined I am to avoid it.

A Strand of Magic in Crisis

Crisis experiences aren't always bad. Sometimes something happens to remind me the magic is still there, it's just hidden. One time I was trying to get through a crisis without going to the hospital. I was in physiological and psychological agony. I decided to walk around in the backyard. For some reason I stopped and looked down. My eyes met with a four-leaf clover towering over the rest of the grass. I had never found a four-leaf clover before. The clover found me. I felt like nature was trying to wish me luck and encourage me to keep going even though I felt hopeless. It felt like everything was dark like psychosis, except for the four-leaf clover popping through.

Another time I was in crisis and pain. I happened to wander into a Starbucks and got a tea. It was getting dark, and I wanted to be inside after spending the day at the park. I had asked the Universe for a sign not too long before because I was struggling, desperate, and suicidal. I was wondering if the Universe was still on my side. I sat in Starbucks longer than I usually ever would and found myself contemplating why I was still there. I was watching videos on my phone when the energy in the room shifted. I felt like something was happening with whoever just entered the store. I looked over and I was right. The Canadian music artist Lights Poxleitner-Bokan, with her signature orange hair, had just walked in the door. I'm not one to get star-struck, but her presence was meaningful. I decided to talk to her. I apologized for bothering her in the traditional Canadian style. I told her I was a big fan and about the times I saw her perform. When I was in the psych ward the first time, when I'd get to go home on a pass, I'd sit and watch the music video for her song "Toes" over and over. I also saw her twice in concert despite not being big on concerts. I told her I was depressed and suicidal and that I asked the Universe for a sign and that she was that sign. "Lights." She was super kind and told me, "It gets better." I asked if we could take a selfie, and she kindly agreed, even having her friend take a few photos. I don't think I could have thought of a better sign from the Universe myself. It was magic. Magic can happen in crisis too. Maybe by watching her repeatedly when I was struggling, I manifested her for real during a future struggle.

One Person's Psychological Thriller is Another Person's Documentary

Movies can play into the scariness too. For a cinematic depiction of interesting angles on death traps, parallel worlds, and suicide, watch *The Discovery* and *Mindgamers*. Warning: these films are psychological/intellectual thrillers and can be triggering. When it feels like something is after me or death is chasing me and my time is running out, psychosis feels like *Final Destination*. Sometimes movies are more real than reality. What I mean is, as an experiencer of mania and psychosis, what they show in movies as fiction are instead real experiences in psychosis. Watching them can lead to my brain remembering how reality is as strange as 'fiction.' Often, we get taken to the hospital before we hurt ourselves or others, because we think that we might. It's a bit like the show *Person of Interest* where "The Machine also identifies perpetrators and victims of other premeditated deadly crimes." When we check in to a psychiatric hospital, it's like we or others are identifying ourselves as persons of interest. We are the victims, possible perpetrators, and heroes. We stop the evil from taking us over, like it has taken over so many. We are turning ourselves in and surrendering.

I watched the film *Momento* and had a long conversation with a friend, trying to figure it out afterward. I slipped into psychosis when I realized that being diagnosed with a mental illness was necessary to maintain myself in consensus reality and that I had in fact created the mental illness myself as a way to come back from a world unrelated to the status quo. I wasn't afflicted with it: I created it, otherwise I'd be in the eternal afterlife. It was necessary to continue as I knew myself to be since I created so many tangent realities in mania and had to face so much karma and collective karma in psychosis. Sometimes psychosis feels like a tangent reality like the movie *Donnie Darko*, where we get some extra time to live as we want in mania, only for that tangent reality to collapse. Imagine saying when mania ends, "Oh that tangent reality died."

As I mentioned earlier, before I went to the psych ward for the first time, I have a memory of choosing to be mentally ill so that I could stay here with my family. They didn't want me to leave the Earth. It wasn't my time. What I haven't elaborated on is how in one possibility, I experienced that I was already dead and erased from their reality from something that happened. Their love pulled me back out of the dark energy/matter dream world, a bit like the movie *What Dreams May Come*. Though I didn't die by suicide, I did unconsciously try to make it look like I was attempting suicide during my first crisis. The mental health system tries to reunite families with those who are lost to this world. We are not lost when we lose ourselves, but we are lost to those who lose us. A mental illness diagnosis was the only way to resolve all the parallel Universes I'd stepped into, all the possibilities they initiated, and come back to life. I created the mental illness to come back from the dead. I remember the parallel reality where I didn't make it through. It was terrifying to realize I died and remember dying, yet still being alive. By remembering death, I paradoxically realized immortality. I had to fight my way through psychosis out of compassion for those who did me in, and if I could make it through to the parallel world where I didn't die, they wouldn't have to go to jail. I had to struggle to get back to my loved ones. The only way back to Earth as we know it was the portal of the mental health system. So, I had to go through it. Though no one helped me fake my death, I did fake my suicide attempt, so much so that I fooled myself. This is a bit like *Fight Club*. I wasn't trying to die in psychosis. I was trying to live in mania. The 2021 film *Bliss* has a crazy-trippy-accurate depiction of parallel realities and the sacrifices and benefits of manifesting in each. For some people, these films are representation of daily life, rather than fantasy. Others watch it on films.

I AM SPIRITUALLY GOING CRAZY, AM I?

"You are designed to make a difference in this world."

- Dhyan Vimal

Years before all this started happening, I studied with an enlightened Master. Years later, in 2011, when all the quantum weirdness started happening, I contacted him to ask what the heck was going on. At times, I thought I was going nuts, and other times I felt enlightened. The gap was very small, and it was hard to tell the difference. I had no guide, though I had a compass. He did give me some pointers, but I've been on my own from there. There comes a time when the Master leaves you to your own devices. Then he says, maybe someday we'll meet as friends. This could be true whether you've met one or not. Here is a small excerpt from our conversation.

Master:

The first thing to investigate and put aside is,

is there a medical condition,

What you are saying sounds like a spiritual thing

But before that can be confirm

One must test everything

Just to be sure

Andrea:

I feel like there is a time realm, and a timeless

And when I have to shift, it feels like death

Or the "I" is time, and feels like death, when there is no thought of the self, it feels timeless

Master:

All this is right,

It's part of the awakening process

But you must not go with it, and let it come to you,

No matter what the experience,

you just watch it,

and let it come to you more

Andrea:

Like heavy and everything slows down

It's like $e=mc^2$

When my energy goes to the lower, I feel heavier

Master:

Yes

That is true

Andrea:

When there is that timeless state

I feel no separation from the other

And when leaving them, it feels like death

And, why did what I write to you disappear?

Master:

Hahahah I live this truth

Master:

Understanding must lead to clarity

Andrea:

I'm confused

Master:

Don't be

Just take it easy and let things come to you

Let all arise

Many times when you force this or try too hard it can cause problems to the brain

All that you are saying is wonderful

Andrea:

I feel like I could be crazy

Master:

But the rest of the understanding will come

It takes time

And if you push you feel like you are going crazy

Andrea:

I feel like I can talk to animals

Master:

This might be so, but don't push

Part
FOUR

Practical Preparedness, Tips, and Tricks

"Men have called me mad; but the question is not yet settled, whether madness is or is not the loftiest intelligence—whether much that is glorious—whether all that is profound—does not spring from disease of thought—from moods of mind exalted at the expense of the general intellect. They who dream by day are cognizant of many things which escape those who dream only by night. In their gray visions they obtain glimpses of eternity, and thrill, in waking, to find that they ahead been upon the verge of the great secret."
- Edgar Allan Poe

Chapter 7

IT WAS ALL JUST A MENTAL ILLNESS!?

MERCY, GRACE, RELIEF, AND DEEP-REST

"All muscles need rest. The brain is no exception. Fields must be alternated. Computers must occasionally be shut down or rebooted. To not do this is to risk injury, poor yields, or damage."

- the Daily Stoic

After all the chaos of mania, psychosis, and crisis, thank God sometimes for the reassurance that "it was all just a mental illness," right? It's a chemical imbalance in the brain. I like to think that too on rare occasion and surrender to the higher power of psychosis. It's helpful after a terrifying, death-defying, psychosis, and crisis. Medication equals mercy when we can't find our way through the labyrinth. Accepting that it's just a mental illness is a way to get back into the mainstream world, just like accepting that Jesus is my savior gets me into heaven.

When we have an intense or prolonged mania and psychosis, our brain may feel like mush for a while. It will be hard to function or do everyday tasks. Our regular functioning can and will come back—and much faster if we don't resist or worry too much about it. See it as a natural process that needs some rest and non-doing. Large doses and numbers of initial medications given in the psych ward are often tapered to a much lower dose and number. With patience and rest, we can adapt to the mainstream world again, need less medication, and the side effects can become minimal. We can even get our creativity back.

I once spoke with Dr. Daniel Fisher, a psychiatrist and person with lived experience of a schizophrenia diagnosis. He said he tells his patients, "The medications buy you time." He said the answer lies in repairing and building relationships.

Sometimes medications can lead to iatrogenic illnesses. Iatrogenic illnesses are problems caused by the medications or treatments themselves.[107] It's the harm and risks that hopefully don't outweigh the benefits. Many people experience more harm than good. Psych meds can have side effects like metabolic syndrome, type 2 diabetes, obesity, and cardiovascular disease.[9,108] Our body can also become addicted to medications, so it becomes near impossible to taper off of them if we want to. We experience iatrogenic withdrawal effects that are called symptoms of our illness. This is used to justify the need for continued treatment with medications with statements like, "see, you need to take medications." Medication maintenance treatment, as it's known, is rarely questioned. I recently had a high cholesterol value on a test and my psychiatrist asked me about my diet. The fact that I eat vegetarian food didn't factor in for him. When I inquired about medication side effects, he indicated the medications weren't a factor. When I went home and looked at the side effects, high cholesterol was a side effect for one of them. The possibility of tardive dyskinesia, or uncontrollable movements, is a side effect for three of the four medications I take. Yikes much!

GRIEVING THE LOSS OF OUR MANIC SELF

"Getting hurt is a form of illness."

- J. Krishnamurti

After psychosis and the crisis, we look back and grieve the loss of the manic energy and the manic way of life. We grieve the possibilities we saw for ourselves and the world. We also grieve the normal person we were before we were diagnosed. Diagnosed and medicated, we don't resemble who we were before our bipolar diagnosis or during the heights of mania. I recall looking in the mirror and being afraid of my own reflection—I had flat affect and I looked scary.

The downward tumble from the peak of mania can happen at any time. It manifests differently for everyone. All our psycho-biorhythms are different. Grieving after mania is not unlike grieving the death of a loved one. We loved our manic self. Heck, though we didn't feel it at the time, now we even love our normal self in comparison to our medicated and diagnosed self. Recovering from the downward turn is a bit like the well-known seven stages of grief, though perhaps in a different order. Like the seven states of grief, these can happen in any order when recovering from a crisis:

1) *Pain and anger*

2) *Shock, fear, and denial*

3) *The downward turn*

4) *Guilt and bargaining*

5) *Depression, rejection, and loneliness*

6) *Acceptance and hope*

7) *Reconstruction and work through*

8) *Testing*

In my experience, when pain and anger mix with manic or psychotic energy, bodily sensations can be intense and explosive. Anger can happen in mania due to a sense of entitlement from things not going our way or happening fast enough. Anger can also be directed at the past. If we get angry at the past, the past has infected the present moment, and the manic creative energy is tainted. This is what happens more and more as we go from the euphoria of mania to predominantly psychosis. It's a lose-lose situation and a trick to waste manic energy. The creative energy becomes destructive. Destruction is also necessary for creation; destroying the known to make way for the unknown. It can also destroy relationships. Becoming angry is mediocre, so it helps to fuel the return.

At some point, there is a shock, either when we realize the loss of our presence or when we go too far in our exploration. It's time to turn back. We can't turn back time and avoid the shock that turns us back. It's too late. So, there is nothing we can do once the shock happens. Denial won't help either. We may try certain behaviors to see if we can buy ourselves more time in mania, but we see that no matter which way we turn, it's impossible. Psychosis is a state of dwindling possibilities. It sabotages what is built in mania.

The sabotage is fear. We know when it's over. There's nothing we can do. The downward turn is accompanied by states of mind and behaviors that are low energy, which only serve to further de-energize us. We may feel guilty and bargain with the Universe, but it doesn't respond to begging—only the ego does. As a side effect, the ego is trying to take over control of the brain through the back door. These states are lower than our prior-to-mania egoic state. We are turning ourselves in. As punishment, the ego may try to kill us for attempting to live without it. We are no longer a good host to its parasitic memes. When we bargain, we are trying to energetically make a deal with the ego and all the egos of the constellation we deserted. We agree to be mental patients since that's the main way to re-assimilate and make sense of any disturbance we caused to the false peace of others. The system is the portal back to the mainstream. It's super depressing when we find out that the only way to come back, the mental health system, will get us rejected by those who we endeavor to come back for. Lonely times may follow from rejection to being estranged from our manic self. We start grieving the loss of wholeness. When we accept our new life, there is time to restructure our life and work through the challenges. We can try out and test out new things and see what works for us and start the upward turn. We live the next cycle of our journey up through the levels of consciousness and back again.

ANGER, PAIN, FEAR, AND SHAME

"Go into it - it has some significance (the pain) and that significance depends on each one."

- J. Krishnamurti

Do we become patients because we are not patient? Does this behavior help me become the person psychiatry sees me as? Or become the old me others know me as? Any energy that is shunted to increase private hurts, anger, or judgment destroys the brain cells. We are hurting our brains when we hurt ourselves or others. We need to know what not to do with manic energy as it doesn't belong to us. It's not personal but universal. We can't build a self out of it, or it will only self-destruct through inflation. Look at how what we build in the manic state gets destroyed. Figure out what it is that you must not do because it damages your brain and sabotages the energy. The energy can't abide in a brain lost in the lower ego structures. As sure as the energy can build a new grandiose ego, it can implode upon itself.

Anger springs us backwards. We can even use our new sense of generosity and altruism in mania as an excuse to be angry. Anger in psychosis is worse. We need to learn to drop our anger and hate as they lead to hitting the wall. We need to slip gently past the concept of evil, like Jesus said. Grandiosity is sprinkled with anger and hate. None of the 'energy' can be used for personal gain as what is gained personally is nothing. We can get angry at how slow and 'dumb' people seem to be compared to us in mania, only to be humbled with hitting the wall and becoming even slower and dumber than we've ever been. We may have to shrink at times and humble ourselves so that others don't feel insecure around us. We can learn to do it consciously, or our experience will do it for us. We have to understand our anger to move beyond the violence of it. It sabotages us. It disembodies us. We lose the control stick and start acting out a program.

The Universe tests us to see if we'll harm others for any reason—and the Universe sees all. We must learn not to act based on thought or believe thought. Whether we are told to by another person, by a voice, or by an inner impulse, don't fall for it or you fall into a trap. Thought is not a good reason. Thought is full of bad reasons to believe. There's never a good reason to hurt someone. In my experience, it's best to sit in a fetal position, wait it out, and ask for help. How we will be treated in the psych ward will be much kinder if we freeze and accept help. Then they have to bring us in for "thinking we might hurt someone," which isn't a crime. Hurting someone is a crime. Sometimes we act out because it's the only way to get help, because you have to be so close to hurting yourself or someone else to get help. Tell them clearly it's an emergency, and you are going to hurt someone or yourself if that's how you feel, before you hurt yourself. Wait for them to come get you. Don't be tricked. I also take PRN's.

Thoughts can be neutralized. The fearful thought, "She knows too much," can be negated with "I don't know anything." What is your scariest thought or realization when you shift into psychosis? Try to negate the confusion with the realization that we know nothing. Or make up your own negation statement. If we are patient, we will see that what the scary thoughts say don't come to pass. We only make it come to pass with our fear reaction. If we act or react to the thought, we fulfill the intention of thought to trick us into acting out an illusion. It's like bully games on the playground. The normal state of 80% negative thoughts is just as harmful, though less intense. We are lucky when we notice the tricks of thought because we are one step closer to the truth. If fear takes over, it's temporary. Freeze and wait it out. Don't act it out. When we don't act it out and let is pass, it dies. Truth wins. These negative thought-forms are looking for a host. When we refuse to host them, they give up. They can only live on through us. Each one we allow to pass through us without believing it or acting on it deletes it from the karma of humanity. This is our power. The fear in psychosis is also used to find a portal back to consensus reality. The journey through the psych system is a portal from quantum consciousness to Newtonian consciousness. Psych wards are re-education camps. I'd rather be educated by a Shaman, but it is what it is.

We already have lots of time served. We have lots of practice in a state of fear while feeling like our life is in imminent danger. We have practice in an emergency state of psychosis and an urgency state of mania. When we live through altered states, it's an incredible feat of strength. We can still say we have strength and courage, but to live in altered states, not have a mental illness. There are benefits to getting through urgency and emergency states. It could be practice for future possibilities. We won't panic when the powers that be try to induce panic. There will be a time when such a panic will be induced, and people will run to their deaths—maybe with an alien invasion or one of those "this is not a test" messages we get on our phones. When we aren't afraid of being afraid, we can act intelligently in a fluidly relaxed state. And when you can process that much fear you can process that much ecstasy.

When I see too much and go too far into mania, re-experiencing old trauma and my own evil brings me down many notches. My own trauma scares me back to Earth. Getting scared shitless is one way I go from zoomed out to infinite possibilities to zoomed back into my finite body. When we are grandiose, we will be humbled. It's a safety mechanism so we don't get lost in prophecy. My brain reframes experiences most often shrouded in the shame of labels spouted from the lips of those who've undoubtedly not yet had their brains sprained by the games of the consensus cage. Peace.

DON'T FORGET THE PHYSICAL WORLD

"Make your pain pay you back."

- Gabyland YouTube Channel

Teal Swan said, "Negating the physical dimension with higher truths" is a problem for people on a spiritual path. It's referred to as a spiritual bypass. We can get trapped by this in bipolar too. We can use mania to think we are above certain things like showering, sleeping, eating, or even gravity. We forget Maslow's hierarchy of needs. Honoring the physical dimension provides grounding and a solid reference point. The physical dimension can be used as a control stick that can slow us down when we speed up too much.

First and foremost, we need to take good care of our body and ourselves, for our own sake. The body responds when we take care of it, and we automatically feel better about ourselves.

We are more courageous and confident. If we don't care for our body first, who will? Secondly, it's an unfortunate truth that other people are likely to notice what's not quite right about us. If we look like we're not taking care of ourselves and our body, we're more likely to be treated like crap. If we ignore this, we will experience more perceived "stigma." They can't see our hearts, only our appearance, and humans are programmed to make quick judgments. We can use this to our advantage and spare ourselves a lot of grief by taking care of ourselves when we can. We need to put ourselves first. A mental health diagnosis can be a disguise and excuse for hiding our true powers, but we don't have to hide away from life. When we look good for ourselves, we are not hiding our mental illness, we are disguising our superpowers. We can work towards looking good and disguising our superpowers, but not by trying to remain hidden and invisible. Life needs us to try. It took me six months of grieving the loss of my former self before I started to go out into the community.

Also, doctors are less likely to keep our medications high if we look well. They only have 15 minutes to spend. They are looking us up and down in addition to asking their questions. They'll give us just enough meds to disguise our superpowers, and not keep us in a powerless stupor. Keeping my medication doses low has been key in my wellness journey. I've kept my weight between 105 pounds and 135 pounds. I'm usually about 125 pounds. You can't tell I have a diagnosis, and I can tell you I have superpowers. Other patients in the psych ward have even insisted I was a nurse.

I recommend going to a thrift store and buying some nice clothes that fit well. Don't buy any with holes or stains. I remember how in the very beginning, it was like climbing Mount Everest to do the simplest thing. At first, I only showered, changed into clean clothes, and brushed my teeth every five days. When I took a good look at my face for the first time in several months, I had to use tweezers to pick off some crusted green goop that accumulated at the base of my eyelashes. Initially I only fit into a couple stretchy pants because I'd gained 50 pounds from the medications. I lost a bunch of weight by tracking my food intake in an app, eating healthier food, and exercising a bit. Then, I bought some clothes that I felt good in. I was sheltered by the mental health community at first, then when I ventured out further, I never experienced stigma and I was open about my diagnosis.

We must respect our bodies as they are our spaceship in the Universe. Here are a few examples of what helped me weather the tough times. Some of them are very basic but can be difficult after being diagnosed.

- Eat healthy
- Sleep lots
- Shower/Shave
- Brush teeth
- Floss
- Deodorant
- Clean clothes
- Light makeup
- Pluck eyebrows
- Avoid medications that cause weight gain disproportionate to food intake

- Buy nice clothes for everyday wear that fit well

- Wear a smile too

- Make eye contact

- Say hi to people

- Be polite

- Check-in on posture while sitting and standing

- Practice random acts of kindness

- Don't take life too seriously

- Have self-compassion

- Laugh at oneself

- Don't internalize the stigma game

- …

I'm not a smoker but I always remember a tip from the documentary film called *E-Motion*. Eating a combination of licorice and walnuts helps quit. Smoking will drain your financial resources and put you in the "at risk of dying 25 years early" with a mental illness category.

I find it helpful to clean up my living space often to avoid the impulse to go on a cleaning spree. I put the dishes in the dishwasher, run it, and empty it. I keep up with my laundry. I make sure to feed myself. There's definitely a bipolar hierarchy of needs. The new higher capacities that we've self-actualized don't negate the physical dimension. People won't listen to us if we look unkempt. If we get upset because someone treated us poorly, we can waste precious energy ruminating for days. It may seem like a lot of energy and effort, but it saves energy over time.

The more we can practice all this daily stuff, the more likely we won't ignore it the next time when we are in mania. Sometimes it's impossible to do the most basic things, and that's okay too. And it's okay to ask for help from supporters.

Some of the depressive feelings can be helped by paying attention to posture. Power poses like those presented by Amy Cuddy in her famous TED talk, "Your body language may shape who you are"[109] might also help to mitigate some of the bodily collapse that happens when depression hits. Depression makes gravity feel stronger. Pay attention to how you hold your body when you're depressed versus energetic. Holding an energetic posture despite being depressed is a way of changing our state of mind through embodied cognition. We consciously choose our body posture, and the mind is more likely to give us a mood, or spirit that follows suit. Once in the psych ward I felt this strong negativity pulling me down. In response, I would forcefully adjust my posture and sit up straight. I refused to give in and sit slumped. I had also been put on a high dose of antipsychotics against my will. I knew it could make me rapidly gain weight, so I decided to only to eat half my food at mealtime. I also felt super suicidal and didn't think I was going to pull through. Yet I still made gestures to come through it as best as I could. The Universe knew I wanted to live by my life-affirming gestures. Remember we can use our body intelligence in crisis and in recovery to change our state.

When I was manic for the first time, I made a mess. I had unanswered emails, missed appointments, and tons of purchases. I bought numerous Groupons some had expired while others hadn't. I wanted to salvage what I could from what I'd done. I made a big list and slowly worked through the to-do's one by one. It felt satisfying to address them with a level head. Making lists and crossing things off helps with practicality and yields a hit of dopamine. Adding tasks and events in my calendar and deleting them when finished is the best way to remember what I plan to do.

Make an affirmation that can be said internally or to someone if you feel that you may react and cause conflict, including situations of perceived stigma. Instead of reacting defensively, we can make a positive statement of truth about ourselves. If someone said to me, "What are you doing with your life?" or "You're doing everything wrong," I wouldn't defend myself but affirm myself: "I'm a shiny, sparkly human being. I bring joy to lots of people, and I can't be convinced otherwise." This feels true to me, especially since I've created so much meaningful context to rest upon. I realize they can't know me more than I can, especially since I continue to expand my understanding. Feel free to create your own affirmation.

Lastly, grounding, Earthing, forest bathing, human touch, sunlight, and communing with nature are free. Get as creative as you can about practicality and the physical dimension. We can strengthen the physical dimension with physical truths.

CREATIVE SAFETY FOR WALKING BETWEEN WORLDS

"Working on our own consciousness is the most important thing that we are doing at any moment, and being love is the supreme creative act."

- Ram Dass

I think a lot about how to keep myself safe from myself when I dissociate into suicidal patterns in psychosis. I think a lot about suicide; about how NOT to end my life by suicide. I've created safety plans with redundancies to protect me from myself when I experience incoherence and confusion between my body and mind, good and evil. Do you have a plan to stay alive? I'm really interested in designing safety into my life so I can continue to live my life and attempt to thrive, instead of living in fear of attempting suicide. By succeeding in creating safety, I'm less likely to succeed in destroying my body. I have more to do here, and planning helps to ensure that the end of my story won't be by my own hand.

Know what your rhythms and patterns are. Know when a treatment is making you worse and speak up right away, otherwise it will be called worsening of your illness. We need to be creative and know how to get helpful treatment and help ourselves when we can too. We need to participate in creating that the treatment benefits outweigh the risks. Can we move towards a transformation-friendly mental health system? In the meantime, here are a few ideas to creatively enhance your sense of safety—to feel safe to live your life to the full.

- Fill out your Medical ID app on your iPhone and emergency contacts.

- Know that you can use Siri to call emergency services.

- Know the shortcut buttons on your phone to call emergency or activate Emergency SOS feature on your specific device. This sends your location to all your emergency contacts in your Medical ID app as well as calling emergency services, depending on your configuration.

- Have crisis line phone numbers favorited in your phone.

- Have a crisis plan, Ulysses Agreement, or Advance Directive, Representation Agreement (so trusted supporters can speak on your behalf if you are in the hospital), and perhaps trusted Power of Attorney.

- Download the WRAP app and fill out the sections.

- Get a medical ID bracelet with your diagnosis on it and an emergency contact.

- Know how to keep yourself safe or ground yourself if you get a wave of panic or psychosis that makes you dissociate or lose control.

- Know what medications are helpful and not helpful in a crisis in the psych ward or for calming yourself to avoid the hospital.

- Carry water filtration straws so that you can survive on river water if you run off somewhere.

- Carry your phone and a charging cable and/or solar charger.

- Have a wilderness survival app in your phone that doesn't rely on WIFI or cellular data.

- Know where a peer respite is.

- Use black-out blinds to create a totally dark sleeping environment—a few studies show being in a totally dark room for a greater portion of the day helps mania.[f]

- Mantak Chia says staying in total darkness for 7 days creates DMT and is transformative to help kundalini

Psychosis: https://realization.org/p/mantak-chia/most-effective-cure-for-kundalini-psychosis.html

- Orange lensed glasses can help to block out blue light when using devices, allowing melatonin to be created for restful sleep.[9]

- To stay alert, inhale more than you exhale. To relax, extend your exhale. See more at five minutes: "You'll never be stressed again" https://youtu.be/rzbe1ix2AuM

- Explore med-free alternatives.

- Design your living space as a sanctuary with wellness tools within arm's reach.

- Community building lowers suicide.

- Know the gestures that make you feel safe. I used to carry around a zap strap in case I dissociated and might attempt to kill myself. That way I could keep my body safe, like the handcuffs did. In what way can you intervene to make yourself feel safe?

- I haven't needed to try this tip yet, but it's too simple not to include it and leave it hidden in the science. Keep in mind it can make you dizzy so you need another person to help and make sure you're lying down. I plan to try it next time I'm manic. Ice cold water in the left ear decreases mania. After the vertigo passes, the half of the brain opposite the chilled ear increases activity. Cold caloric stimulation of the left ear (activating the right hemisphere) might temporarily reduce the symptoms of mania, while depression might be temporarily reduced by cold right ear caloric stimulation.[h] It can reduce delusions and other symptoms for 20-60 minutes.[j]

- Don't try to fly.

In an email from Steven Kotler with the subject: Flow Tip #7–Altering Your Perception for Creativity, he mentions the following tool–The Rapid Nasal Breath:

> *This tool falls into Dr. Huberman's second category, it's something we can do to mitigate the stress response after it's already been activated. You'll want to use this right after you feel a surge of stress.*
>
> *Here's how it works:*
>
> *Take a long, deep breath in through your nose. When it feels like you can't breathe any more air in, rapidly sniff as hard as you can. What'll happen is the alveoli in your lungs will snap open, increasing oxygenation and activating the parasympathetic branch of the nervous system.*

For a book full of evidence-based possibilities, see *Choices in Recovery: 27 Non-Drug Options for Adult Mental Health – an Evidence-Based Guide* by Craig Wagner. If you need more support in brainstorming tools and mastering bipolar, there is a unique course. It's about learning how to be bipolar by becoming comfortable with higher intensities for longer durations while maintaining the ability to act "IN Order" in a stepwise manner.

Bipolar In Order

www.bipolaradvantage.com

I also recommend:

WRAP or Wellness Recovery Action Plan
https://www.wellnessrecoveryactionplan.com

Bipolar or Waking up video series:

https://www.youtube.com/user/bipolarorwakingup

There are tips from an article by Dr. Michael Cornwall, "Responding to Madness with Loving Receptivity: A Practical Guide."[110] If you are struggling with your family relationships and don't think they can be repaired, there is a book about that: "Breaking from Your Parents" by Daniel Mackler. For me, it's important for me to remember to be a good family member when some states can cause me to temporarily forget. If you want to know what else you can do when you've created safety for yourself, read *Own our Own* by Judi Chamberlin. She was institutionalized for years, and her story is incredible.

If you have a strong desire to explore tapering off medication, here are a few resources to consider with the support of your psychiatrist, if possible. Will Hall said The Harm Reduction approach considers that there are risks to coming off medications as well as risks to staying on them. This means we may need to find a doctor who supports our decision to become free of medications or other supporters. I tapered off for five months with the Hardy Nutritionals micronutrients only to end up back on meds. It was worth it to me to know that it's possible to be off them sometimes. There's nothing like falling asleep naturally without a tranquilizer. Thousands of us have tapered off, including Aspen Morrow who wrote the book *Med Free Bipolar*. She takes micronutrients, just like I did. She found some additional clues that I hope will lead me to success next time I try. For now, I've learned that I can adapt to medications, enjoying the benefits and minimizing most of the side effects, besides low libido and oversleeping. Safer medication tapering possibilities:

The Harm Reduction Guide to Coming Off Psych Drugs:

http://willhall.net/comingoffmeds/

The Withdrawal Project: Are you thinking of coming off psychiatric drugs?

https://withdrawal.theinnercompass.org

Naturopath with bipolar Dr. Peter Smith uses Remedies, Vitamins, and Supplements:

balancingbrainchemistry.co.uk

His website has tons of information.

Tapering off Meds with Micronutrients Phone Support:

www.hardynutritionals.com

www.truehope.com

Medication Tapering Coach:

www.chayagrossberg.com

Look at Eva Edelmen's book *Natural Healing for Bipolar Disorder: A Compendium of Nutritional Approaches.*

www.boragebooks.com

Water is important. The book *Your Body's Many Cries for Water* by Dr. Fereydoon Batmanghelidj says the following:

- *The brain function takes absolute priority over all the other systems. The brain is about two per cent of the total body weight, but it receives 18 to 20 per cent of blood circulation.*

- *The various signals produced by these water distributors are indicators of regional thirst and drought of the body. At the onset, they can be relieved by an increased intake of water, yet they are improperly dealt with by the use of commercial chemical products until pathology is established and diseases are born. This error continues with the use of more and more chemicals to treat other developing symptoms, the complications of dehydration become unavoidable, and then the patient dies. The irony of this is that the practitioners say the patient died of a disease! [111]*

In a study, Dehydration Influences Mood, Cognition, they state:

- *Drinking plenty of water is particularly important for those of us with bipolar disorder, because many of the medications we take cause side effects, such as dry mouth or dehydration, which result from frequent trips to the bathroom.*

- *Dehydration changes our mood, so we don't want to do anything (until we drink some water?)*

- *At the moment, the dry mouth is the only accepted sign of dehydration of the body. As I have explained, this signal is the last outward sign of extreme dehydration.[112]*

This chapter isn't meant to be an exhaustive list, but a head start. The list of possible tools is endless, but you need to experiment to find what exactly works for you.

Chapter 8

MORE HINTS FOR NAVIGATING THE NEXT TIME

HEDONISM HARM REDUCTION

"The most important thing is this: to be willing at any moment to sacrifice what we are for what we can become."

- Charles Du Bois

My first mania was extreme and ended in extreme psychosis. I spend hundreds of dollars at thrift stores and on Groupons. I gave cash away to homeless people. I signed up to sponsor a child. I spent $3,000 at the Apple Store in one day on a MacBook Air and iPhone. I signed up to have organic produce delivered. Mania and instant gratification don't mix. We must learn this lesson—the sooner the better. When we grasp this, we won't repeatedly drain our bank account or rack up credit card debt. I've learned to curb hedonism and overspending. If I have a bit of mania, I spend a little bit more, but I buy things I need on my 'to buy' radar.

The pleasure-seeking ego structure is built on "hedonic adaptation" or the need for more and more pleasure, and to decrease pain. The energy of mania can elevate hedonism to new extremes. The mind is programmed to hedonism to drive the economy. Our whole life can easily be designed around the endless consumption of pleasures like food, sex, and entertainment. Besides, what else is there? Magic. The energy of mania can show us how much more there is to life. At the same time, mania can augment our hedonistic programming. What's the problem with too much pleasure? If we eat a tub of ice cream, it tastes good when we eat it, but we suffer later. When we have a long hedonistic mania, we crash and burn. In mania, we may experience too much magic, but magic and hedonism don't mix. We conjure more risks to get more pleasure.

According to Healthline, bipolar can lead to drug and alcohol use, spending sprees, and an unrealistic belief in our own abilities.[113] Mania is deliverance—being set free. Psychiatry is deliverance—being rescued. We're not ready to be set free for good. To be free takes disciplined learning and isn't a license to increase hedonistic activities. Mania is to learn to be in harmony with all of creation, not to create our own fleeting pleasures. It is nice to be recused from our mistakes by psychiatry, but it also silences us from talking about what our experience means. If all there is to mania is hedonism, then psychiatry is right—it doesn't mean much at all. Focusing on hedonistic activities gives bipolar a bad name. Or, if bipolar is mainly hedonism, certainly some of us would like to go beyond it to human potential. Maybe some of us have bipolar with hedonistic features and others don't. I don't identify with the typical hedonistic categories. There are alternative ways to channel manic energy.

Mania feels like our body is unlocked, uninhibited, and there is no right or wrong. We seek reward through extreme and risky behaviors. We create nightmares that we can't wake up from. So how do we want to live with these states and in these states? Do we need repeated monkey mind pleasures, or can we make a qualitative and quantitative shift? Unless we want the Universe to keep chewing us up and spitting us out, experiment with dropping hedonism. Don't pursue pleasure. Try to channel the energy into something other than the stereotype. If you can, make health and nature your hedonism instead. Behold beauty and create joy instead of hedonism. If we spend our extra cash on vitamins during our next mania, art supplies, or a new computer to write a book, we're on the right track. If we spend it on alcohol and drugs, we're off.

I paint hedonism in a negative light because hedonism and grandiosity are processes that inflate the ego. We are feeding the ego and making it more important with our actions. Ego inflation is a necessary part of the mania sabotage mechanism. If we channel the energy of mania into hedonism, it'll result in ego inflation and self-sabotage to bring us back down to Earth. It's a failsafe. Even if mania goes on for an extended period without hedonism, we can still reach cortical limits for that iteration of mania, and the iteration ends. In plain terms, reaching cortical limits is the brain stretching as far as it can before it runs out of resources. If mania unfolds mainly hedonistically, the cortical limits of the potential of that iteration will not be met. Without hedonism, we will meet the cortical limits of the iteration of mania and return to a lower energy state. Will we learn something new in the next iteration of mania, and soar to new cortical heights? Or will we keep shunting the energy to hedonism and trivial pleasures, rather than building new neural networks through neuroplasticity. Perhaps there's an inverse relationship between the amount of energy wasted on hedonism and the ground we can cover exploring the unknown. The further we go into the unknown, the more likely we are to experience a necessary crisis or psychosis to return. The further we go into the known, or hedonism, the more likely we are to experience a necessary crisis or psychosis to return. It's the same ends, but a totally different means and experience.

THE PITFALLS OF EGO INFLATION AND GRANDIOSITY

"Learning through rewards is more effective
than learning through pain."

- A Course in Miracles

An email I got from the Daily Stoic on March 4th, 2020, said, "Courage becomes a fault when we begin to endanger ourselves and others." Up until that moment, I'd never thought of mania in those terms—as having courage to a fault. Is it courage to a fault that gives us the confidence to carry out our mission? Is our apparent recklessness courage to a fault? Do we have an inflated sense of courage when we drive too fast? Are we courageous when it's unnecessary to be courageous, like if we strip butt-naked and run down the street? That takes courage. Are we making up for moments that we failed to be courageous? Are we wasting our courage? What will happen if we can tone down unnecessary courage? Will we be less likely to be captured and re-educated by psychiatry if we don't run naked down the street? Is this courage part of an inflated ego or a liberated soul? Is courage a fault when coupled with grandiosity?

In the book *1000: The Levels of Consciousness and a Map of the Stages of Awakening for Spiritual Seekers and Teachers* by Ramaji with Ananda Devi,[114] they address the challenge of ego inflation that can happened with spiritual growth up through the levels of consciousness, towards enlightenment and becoming a spiritual teacher. Ramaji's pointers extrapolate to the grandiosity that can happen in mania. He mentions buying into being a "more than human character" where we eventually claim to be the equivalent of God. We find that we've gone farther than we can handle.

The book *1000* is not about mania or bipolar, but it shows mania has similar traps to spiritual growth. Many of us experience mania as extremely spiritual. Ramaji points out that it's easy to fall into the trap of self-inflation and fall back down the levels of consciousness. To Carl Jung, inflation is a response to spiritually being in a position of elevation, influence, and power that you aren't prepared for.[114] The first time in mania, we aren't prepared for the power, elevation, magnetism, and influence we have. People on a spiritual path know about the ego and not to let it get in the way, yet they can still fall for it. Mania is an elevation, and our mental models rearrange, and the ego can inflate along with it. We can be totally unprepared in our first mania, having no context or wisdom tradition. No wonder we always fall for the traps of the ego. In spiritual circles and society, constant upward progress is the ideal. Ramaji illustrates that consistent, linear, upward progress isn't the only way, and that even those close to being teachers of enlightenment can fall into a trap. There are traps and mechanisms that can lead to us falling backward, whether in mania or as a spiritual teacher. It's not wrong or a failure or illness. It's a possibility of the path and part of the learning process. If a spiritual teacher falls, they can learn from their mistake and rise again. We too need to rise again after each time we fall.

The ego-self doesn't know it's not needed in the higher states because it has no real awareness. It continues to try to involve itself in everything and make everything like itself. In mania, we take parts of the ego where it doesn't belong and where it's not designed to go. We haven't done the work to rid of its rule. The ego is not meant to leave the past and go into higher states of consciousness, which are qualitatively future states of consciousness. When we leave the past, we are in the future, and the future is now. The now is actually the future relative to the ego. If we drop the ego, we are in the future now. Take this another step and if many of us did this together, we would 'time travel' to a future world now. Nothing would happen. The real would appear.

Ramaji says we need to be prepared for elevation, and only we can prepare ourselves. After mania, we can begin to prepare for the next mania, or elevation, through Self-dialogue. I mentioned in an earlier chapter the importance of not believing anything. Ramaji reminds us especially to not believe our own hype. There is a difference between experiencing our own hype and believing it. Experiencing it makes it pass while believing it creates a story of importance. Mania often leads to proclaiming that we are Jesus, Mother Theresa, Buddha, etc. This is a clue that mania is a path towards enlightenment, or a propulsion into the state of enlightenment for which we are unprepared and have little context to reference. In mania we go astray because we don't understand the purpose of the energy or territory of enlightenment. It has nothing to do with who we thought we were, or who we think we are when we are feeling enlightened.

Even Ramaji says there is no help to deal with these challenges in spiritual teachings. The same traps and pitfalls that happen on the spiritual path are the pitfalls that swallow people into the mental health system. Is that why Joseph Campbell said that "The psychotic drowns in the same waters in which the mystic swims with delight?" Imagine if we had enough spiritual, Shamanistic, or human potential context in our brains beforehand. We would have a better chance at avoiding psychiatric engulfment. So, we must figure it out for ourselves. Take note, it's normal to go astray, fall backward, and experience discontinuity instead of perfect, ever-increasing linear growth. It's okay to leap way ahead of what you're ready for according to a slow linear path. Maybe some of us are meant to be spiritual teachers? Can we help each other embody the roles we are creating for ourselves, whether it be teacher, painter, channeler, or psychic?

In my case, I wasn't at a level of consciousness where I was trying to be a spiritual teacher. I felt like I was on a spiritual journey, and I was trying to learn along the way. I got to a point where I felt like Jesus. I didn't really think I was Jesus, and even though I wasn't raised religious, I felt connected to him. I thought, "I must feel like he must have felt." I experienced that I had some of the same powers and more, just as he said. Mania is a level more powerful than Jesus. In mania, you know you can do what Jesus said…this and more you shall do. He said we can do more, and we do more in mania. Mania is actually listening to Jesus and living what he said. I took on the Christian lens for a time. I felt like I literally understood what the bible said, even though I've never read past the first page. It wasn't theoretical, the information was in my DNA, and I could see what the bible was saying everywhere. The wisdom of the bible overlaid my reality and augmented it. I tried to act according to it. I felt like maybe I was experiencing Christ Consciousness. I wondered if I was part of the "Christification of many." Whether any of that was true or not, in that state I felt like it was. It didn't last long. Rather than a permanent state of being, it felt like a passing possible reality. I felt fortunate to tap into it, even if it was fleeting. It was like putting on JC glasses to understand what enlightenment was like. I can still feel the afterglow, and to me, that afterglow has tremendous value.

In mania, we do feel "superhuman" and "more than human." We more than feel it, we embody it and live it, subjectively and objectively for a time. It's as if we live in a different time period altogether. We aren't a consistent, linear entity like we've been taught. We are what we act in the situation. We are the situation, and we can situate. They say, "You are what you eat," and "You are what you say." If we are what we act, then being spontaneous improvisation based on and with the actuality of the moment is of the highest value. Our body is physically stronger. Since we are able to perform at a high level, we naturally try higher level actions and experiences.

Don't get attached to mania. It's temporary, nontemporal, nonlinear. It's "non" most things we know. Feel the grandeur of interconnection and oneness. It's eternally and infinitely alive. Don't get grandiose in thinking we are above and outside of life. We are all of life from high to low. We see it's true after reaching a height and get humbled to the low. We go from enlightenment down to shame, only to climb to enlightenment again. There is no time, only consciousness. Do we have a loss aversion reaction to the ending of the manic state? We resist, kicking and screaming. We need to freeze to make the rise humbler and the tumble softer. We have to learn how to humble ourselves or the mental health system will do it for us. Perhaps realizing that mania is a state that is superior to the less energetic manifestations of ourselves rather than being superior to others will save us some grief.

Don't believe anything beyond a moment. It's an interesting or insightful perception in awareness, not a thing to be believed in. Truth only applies to the moment it arises in. Truth is infinite. No belief is required, only witnessing attention. When you don't believe, you'll apprehend what is. You'll avoid creating stories and a storyteller by stringing together beliefs. Undo the belief in the believer. Unbelievable things will occur to you, then drop it. This is not only a safety and survival issue, but a recognition and acknowledgement that there is so much more that can arise in an empty container in the very next moment. You are an empty channel for bringing new information into the known Universe, not a self to believe and become full of what it identifies as itself. That's wasting attention. The quote on my Yogi Tea brand tea once said, "Empty yourself and let the Universe fill you."

Back to the assumption in many spiritual circles that any spiritual or human potential growth must be linear and consciously earned. This is the same assumption in society about how humans learn and grow. Mania shows the assumption isn't true and that we can spring forward to consciously unearned states of higher consciousness. We can mutate and transform and, conversely, we can revert to the ego again. That's what Trans-Consciousness is. In the acceptable time-bound mechanism, the ego can consciously, slowly, and progressively deconstruct itself. Large jumps are seen as illness because we don't realize we are consciousness, not a self. Since the ego is not existential, it can disengage in an instant. It follows that existence, or the Universe can show us instantly that the ego is unreal, and we'd instantly transform. Existence takes the place of nonexistence in a moment. One is the present; the other is the past. Immediate, radical transformation induced by the Universe is whole and complete. The instantaneous mutation process is real. A problem in the recovery movement is that the status quo is promoted as real when anyone who goes into the manic realm knows that realm is more real. It's existence. The Universe shifts us back to tell others, but they won't listen. We must take a stand and declare that our instant mutation process is also human potential and transformation, not human illness. We may be majorly shaken up when we shift back to mainstream, not because we were in a trance, but because we returned to the consensus trance. Mania is a big leap forward, and psychosis is a big leap back. Both have costs but they also have benefits. Depression is a reaction to being in the illusion. Ramaji says he knows of no course to help with the challenges of inflation and hype and fall back.

ON BEING POWERFUL IN PROGRAMMED PLACES, TRIPPING ON GRACE, AND CUSHIONING THE FALL ON YOUR FACES

"With great power comes great responsibility."

- Voltaire, and Uncle Ben from Spiderman

The gift and the challenge of being touched with fire are that we can really feel and see things, perhaps as if for the first time since we were young kids. Everything feels so new. We are also infants in the sense that we are interacting with so many new parts of reality that we couldn't see before. Humans exploring the unknown is in its infancy, and our growth is being stunted. We are infants to our new senses, abilities, and powers, and we have no one to hold our hand while we learn to walk. All our known and unknown senses are sensitized, and it can take time to adapt.

In energized states of consciousness, we can apply less "force" to do the same things. Too much force burns out the brain cells. A Karate Master can apply less force to break a board since the force is skillfully directed. Others would injure themselves trying to break the same board. It's helpful to realize that there is a non-doing that does everything. The non-doing is less force as non-doing has more power. Doing is of the ego and is just a piddly recruitment of neurons compared to having the whole Universe on your side. Non-doing employs the powers of the Universe. Try doing nothing when the energy of mania is there, at least for one iteration. One time in mania, all I did was lay on the grass in a park. I experienced that the heightened state wasn't too high, psychosis was manageable, and the low wasn't too low. I had a crisis and didn't need the hospital. Maybe that's why people go meditate in caves, to leave it up to the Universe. It's still working through us when we do nothing or everything we can.

SHIFTING BACK AND FORTH BETWEEN STATES – PHASE TRANSITION AND REVERSE METAMORPHOSIS

"Is this a friendly Universe?"

- Albert Einstein

Mania works and plays best among friendly strangers in the friendly Universe. But what happens when we encounter unfriendliness? Our past world contains our unfriendly ego persona. Our ego is not our friend. People we know have memories and images of us, and they can unknowingly project them onto us when we'd like to imagine we're beyond that version of ourselves. Being shrink-wrapped by the past sucks. It's a buzzkill, and it's hard on the brain. We know that thought projections influence us. They act like a web. Just as we can make the world magical with magical manic consciousness, others can limit us with their projections. We can fall into patterns that they want us to play out. They don't know thought is participatory, so they don't know what they are doing to us. It's the mechanism of mediocrity. In mania, we can see the subtle, and we can see what others are doing unknowingly with their thoughts. It's one thing that creates "disproportionate" outbursts of anger. If the not-so-subtle effects of thinking became perceptible, they'd be criminalized. We can read the thoughts of others and their body language. We can't be criminalized for our thoughts, but we can be psychiatrized.

In mania, we are 'yes-ing'ourselves into being. Anyone who knows us, 'nos' us. We no longer are attracted to being reminded of who we were. The ego makes us seize up when moments before we were flowing freely. Our mood appears to shift rapidly. Energy rapidly decelerates and drops, and we have to time travel and shift backward. Mutating from mania to ego is painful. We do it for others—to comply with their operating system. They are trying to bring us down and assimilate us if they sense we've gone beyond ourselves. We get tricked into shifting back into ego mode to play that game. To shift is compassion. Not to shift is to deny their existence. And they don't exist in the now. We need to get better at shifting and used to the pain. In a lower resonance, the degrees of freedom of action we have are limited to the marionette strings of our conditioning. The constellation limits the combination of ego patterns playing out in a scene. The phase shift from the state of manic flow to interacting with the known past in familiar patterns can be dramatic. Shifting back is often accompanied by a dramatic shift in mood resulting in anger at losing our energetic state. Without a shield, the projections of others can get right through, and we react. Lower energy reaction is part of the mechanism that contributes to the shift back—it's the intelligence of the so-called mood disorder. It's a shift between orders of reality that show as an apparent mood. The "mood-disorder" will still always upshift us back to mania at some point.

FINAL RESONANT COGNITIVE DISSONANCE

*"When you are doing something which you
cannot help doing with your whole being,
you are being yourself."*

- J. Krishnamurti

You are invited to take your power back. The power is the capacity to find out for yourself and make up your own mind—to create yourself from the original blueprint you came with when you were born. Mania gives us a map to that blueprint.

Can mania be normalized so we can live extraordinarily? Through glorification, full acceptance, and attentive awareness, the idea of mania as an illness can be slowly crowded out. We can see it as the creative, healing process that it is, closing the gap between our actual and false being. More people need to let loose and see they already are who they are, and that it's qualitatively different than we think ourselves into being. More normal people need to act a little more manic and magical. Instead of playing false roles, we need to play more for real, in daily life. Why do we have to go back to being normal after mania? Why is the whole world waiting for a reason to be happy for no reason? Being human is not enough, because we don't know what it means to be human. We don't know our true power and possibility.

What if instead of being suppressed and reined in with medications for the comfort of others, we had a license and the qualifications to act differently, out of character, and at times radically nuts so that we are a new being? In mania, something new is trying to come into being through us. What if we could be happy for no reason, not even because of mania? The solution for sanity isn't for me to control myself with meds, but for all of us to stop controlling ourselves with the ego. It's the wrong controller, and it's using our interface and inner face. There's nothing we have to do to make this happen. The energy to be free now is already always available. We can plug in to the infinite source. While we are integrating our experience, we can help others get it.

Maybe our life as we normally think we see it and experience it is the illusion? It's warped by the past. Maybe when see hallucinations, we see the past in place of the present? The past mixes with material reality and warps it so we materially experience what isn't really happening. We make matter bend to our thoughts. We feel heavy because the warped and hallucinated reality is out of alignment with conscious manifestation.

Maybe the past is material substance, and reality is really an eternal quantum dream where energy and information predominate over matter? Maybe matter doesn't matter? Maybe in mania, we are seeing something important? Maybe we are seeing something about the true nature of reality? Physicists say the nature of reality at a very small level is quantum. Do we see the quantum nature of reality? Can these extrapolations and superpositions help us ground mania in our daily lives? Is there anywhere where mania, bipolar, human potential, and the frontiers of science intersect? Maybe the possible future has already happened?

We can build intrapersonal intelligence for ourselves, or how we understand ourselves in light of mania. We can create a linguistic scaffolding for the manic intra-subjective space and some common language that we can draw from. By doing this, we open the dimension of "epi-mania," or control above the level of mania. We could also call it "intra-mania," "meta-mania," or "para-mania" in that we are internally rearranging our blocks of meaning and context with our conscious subjectivity in retrospect and prospect. We can become bipolar "polymaths" or "people of wide knowledge or learning." We can only learn and act our way through, as, in, out, and beyond this. It becomes a self-fulfilling prophecy of fulfilling ourselves. In the end, there are more questions, and rather than doing a scientific study on each, I can ask Gaia and the Universe and get an immediate response. Such is the power of emptiness and the source. These are the keys. These are the connections. When we are empty, we are entangled with all and summon information through direct contact with the quantum field. It'll take science many years and billions of dollars to find out that what we experience is truth speaking to us. We don't have to wait to speak our truth, as a living truth, now. We have to tell ourselves who we are, or we'll keep playing the game of the mental patient. Through our brain, eyes, hands, heart, and voice, we are re-gaming bipolar.

Is this book a sign I wasn't on enough medications to have insight into my illness? Or is it, as Kay Redfield Jamison put in her book, *Touched with Fire - Manic Depressive Illness and Artistic Temperament:*[115]

> *The ethical issues arising from such knowledge, and from the possibility that such a devastating illness can confer individual and societal advantage, are staggering: Would one want to get rid of this illness if one could?*

I know I wouldn't. And remember, no matter what you think you did or done you can find yourself and have fun. If you realize you will learn your way through it, that's all that's needed—the learning will happen. Because you intentionally willed it by realizing you can. It's not impossible. You are possible. 'See willing possibilities' for your exploration.

You are invited to participate...see you in level 2.

Thank you for your precious time and attention.

https://linktr.ee/bipolargamechanger

ACKNOWLEDGMENTS

To my family, I love you so much. Thank you Uday, so many 'brain twin' dialogues over the years gave me permission and support to draft and craft. Nicole you've had a profound impact on my life. Thanks for being a friend and mentor. Anastasia for the bumblebee effect. Dawn and Ginny for friends for life. Ron Unger for allowing me to quote your wisdom liberally. To everyone who's helped me through the mental health system so I could re-discover and re-create my life—doctors, clinicians, workers, peers, members, friends, family groups, acquaintances, and friendly strangers. Thank you to the clubhouse, my second family. Thanks Holly, Ryan, Devon, Monica, James, Anat, Kevin, Michael, and Rafael. To Eckhart Tolle, J. Krishnamurti, Alan Watts, and Dhyan Vimal. To the advocates and paradigm shifters whom I've met briefly in person or via audio or video call or email like Will Hall, Victoria Maxwell, Emma Bragdon, Sean Blackwell, Ron Unger, Dr. Dan Fisher, Dabney Alix, Dr. Peter Smith, Dmitry Gutkovich, the author of "Life with Voices" for supporting me with a disclaimer, and so many more! To all the peer movements and organizations. Thank you Marie Still for editing, J.A. Rapps for the references, via creative for the book design, sam_designs1 for the cover, beta readers medavaitonyte and alvenecus, msgrgr, and other Fiverr creators like nicolecarino. Thank you, synchronicity, for all the special messages. Thank you, Gaia. Thanks to all the authors who wrote the books I've read. Thanks for all the documentaries and their makers. To the music artists Lights and Celine Dion for giving me hope. Electronic music for your beats. Tucker Max at Scribe Media Book School for the free course that sparked me to start writing a book. Thanks, technology, for making self-publishing possible. I want to acknowledge the work of every human being I've quoted, referenced, and extrapolated from beyond their intended context or views, hopefully within the bounds of fair use. You have fortunately inadvertently shed light on the mysteries of mental health transformation. If I have unfortunately gone beyond fair use or fair extrapolation, I offer expressed written forgiveness. My intention is to build bridges to your genius and throw a life ring to those drowning in a sea that, without the help of your discoveries to re-contextualize our living experience, we might otherwise continue to flounder. I am grateful to the human endeavor that moves us to flowering, together. To joyous exploration.

A CHAOS OF REFERENCES

i.   Akiskal, H.S., Azorin, J.M., Hantouche, E.G. Proposed multidimensional structure of mania: Beyond the euphoric-dysphoric dichotomy. *Journal of Affective Disorders.* **73** (1-2), 7–18 (2003).

ii.   Beigel A., Murphy, D.L., Bunney, W.E., Jr. The manic-state rating scale: Scale construction, reliability, and validity. *Archives of General Psychiatry.* **25**, 256–62 (1971).

a.   Alexander, B. K., Coambs, R. B. & Hadaway, P. F. The effect of housing and gender on morphine self-administration in rats. *Psychopharmacology (Berl).* **58**, 175–179 (1978).

b.   DeFehr, J. N. Inventing Mental Health First Aid: The Problem of Psychocentrism. *Stud. Soc. Justice* **10**, 18–35 (2016).

c.   Whitaker, R. The WHO Calls for Radical Change in Global Mental Health. *Mad in America* https://www.madinamerica.com/2021/06/calls-radical-change-global-mental-health/ (2021).

d.   Raviv, S. The Genius Neuroscientist Who Might Hold the Key to True AI. *Wired* https://www.wired.com/story/karl-friston-free-energy-principle-artificial-intelligence/ (2018).

e.   Gepp, K. What the Eyes Can – and Can't – Reveal About Bipolar Disorder. *Healthline* https://www.healthline.com/health/bipolar-disorder/bipolar-eyes (2021).

f.   Barbini, B., Benedetti, F., Colombo, C., Dotoli, D., Bernasconi, A., Cigala-Fulgosi, M., Florita, M. & Smeraldi, E. "Dark Therapy for Mania: A Pilot Study." *Bipolar Disorders.* **7** (1), 98–101 (2005).

g.   Wirz-Justice, A. & Terman, M. Commentary on 'Blue-blocking glasses as additive treatment for mania: a randomized placebo-controlled trial.' *Bipolar Disord.* **18**, 383–384 (2016).

h.   Pettigrew, J. D. & Miller, S. M. A sticky interhemispheric switch in bipolar disorder? *Proc. R. Soc. London. Ser. B Biol. Sci.* **265**, 2141–2148 (1998).

j.   Levine, J. *et al.* Beneficial effects of caloric vestibular stimulation on denial of illness and manic delusions in schizoaffective disorder: a case report. *Brain Stimul.* **5**, 267–273 (2012).

k.   Kaufman, S,B. &. Gregoire, C. "How to Cultivate Creativity: Research shows that being open to new experiences spurs innovation in the arts, sciences and life." *Sci. Am. Mind.* (Jan/Feb 2016)

2.   Hawkins, D. R. *Power vs. Force*. (Hay House Inc., 2014).

3.   American Psychiatric Association. Diagnostic and Statistical Manual of Mental Disorders, Fifth Edition (DSM-5). (2013).

4.   *Psychiatry Disrupted*: Theorizing Resistance and Crafting the (R) evolution. (McGill-Queen's University Press, 2014).

5.   Academy of Ideas. What Happened to Nietzsche? - Madness and the Divine Mania. *YouTube* https://www.youtube.com/watch?v=gjo8EDXGUI0 (2021).

6.   National Institute of Mental Health. Bipolar Disorder. https://www.nimh. nih.gov/health/topics/bipolar-disorder.

7.   Dome, P., Rihmer, Z. & Gonda, X. Suicide Risk in Bipolar Disorder: A Brief Review. *Medicina (B. Aires).* **55**, (2019).

8.   Fortuna, K. L. *et al.* Systematic Review of Behavioral Health Homes Impact on Cardiometabolic Risk Factors for Adults with Serious Mental Illness. *Psychiatr. Serv.* **71**, 57 (2020).

9.   Fava, G. A. & Rafanelli, C. Iatrogenic Factors in Psychopathology. *Psychother. Psychosom.* **88**, 129–140 (2019).

10. Warden, D., Rush, A. J., Trivedi, M. H., Fava, M. & R Wisniewski, S. The STAR*D Project results: a comprehensive review of findings. *Curr. Psychiatry Rep.* **9**, 449–459 (2007).

11. National Hearing Voices Network. https://www.hearing-voices.org/

12. Merriam-Webster. Extrapolate. https://www.merriam-webster.com/ dictionary/extrapolate.

13. *The Essential David Bohm*. (Routledge, 2002).

14. Watson, K. & Browne, D. What Is Synesthesia? *Healthline* https://www. healthline.com/health/synesthesia (2018).

15. Parrish, S. The Map Is Not the Territory. *Farnam Street* https:// fs.blog/2015/11/map-and-territory/ (2015).

16. Krishnamurti, J. Is there thinking without the word? https://jkrishnamurti.

org/content/there-thinking-without-word (1976).

17. Lesson 11. in *A Course in Miracles: Workbook for Students/Manual for Teachers* (eds. Schucman, H., Thetford, B. & Wapnick, K.) (Viking, 1976).

18. Ackerman, C. E. What is Positive Psychology & Why is It Important? *PositivePsychology* https://positivepsychology.com/what-is-positive-psychology-definition/ (2020).

19. Greenwood, T. A. Positive Traits in the Bipolar Spectrum: The Space between Madness and Genius. *Mol. Neuropsychiatry* **2**, 198–212 (2017).

20. Merikangas, K. R. *et al.* Lifetime and 12-Month Prevalence of Bipolar Spectrum Disorder in the National Comorbidity Survey Replication. *Arch. Gen. Psychiatry* **64**, 543–552 (2007).

21. James, M. *A Bipolar Expedition*. (Roast Beef Productions, 2010).

22. Unger, R. CBT for Psychosis. *udemy* https://www.udemy.com/course/cbt-for-psychosis/ (2021).

23. Bodnar, M. The Simple 20 Minute Exercise That Rewires Your Brain For Happiness with Dr. Dan Siegel. *The Science of Success Podcast* https://www.successpodcast.com/show-notes/2019/1/9/the-simple-20-minute-exercise-that-rewires-your-brain-for-happiness-with-dr-dan-siegel (2019).

24. National Geographic. Dark Matter and Dark Energy. https://www.nationalgeographic.com/science/article/dark-matter.

25. Reporters, T. Professor Stephen Hawking's final theory. *Telegraph* https://www.telegraph.co.uk/news/2018/05/02/professor-stephen-hawkings-final-theory-Universe-hologram/ (2018).

26. Ornes, S. News Feature: Quantum effects enter the macroworld. *Proc. Natl. Acad. Sci.* **116**, 22413–22417 (2019).

27. Gardner, J. Patient-centred medicine and the broad clinical gaze: Measuringoutcomes in paediatric deep brain stimulation. *Biosocieties* **12**, 239–256 (2017).

28. Wikipedia. Gaslighting. https://en.wikipedia.org/wiki/Gaslighting.

29. Collins Dictionary. Menticide. https://www.collinsdictionary.com/dictionary/english/menticide.

30. Grof, S. & Bennett, H. Z. The Holotropic Mind: The Three Levels of Human Consciousness and How They Shape Our Lives. (HarperOne, 1993).

31. Krishnamurti, J. *The First Step is the Last Step*. (Krishnamurti Foundation India, 2004).

32. Unger, R. About Ron Unger. *Recovery From schizophrenia* (2009). https://

recoveryfromschizophrenia.org/about-ron-unger/

33.   Antidepressant Discontinuation: The Why & How of Tapering. *Kelly Brogan MD* https://www.kellybroganmd.com/blog/antidepressant-discontinuation-why-and-how.

34.   Unger, R. From Madness to Mastery: Gaining Competence with Altered States. *Recovery From schizophrenia* (2017).

35.   Unger, R. Spiritual Issues Within Treatment for Psychosis and Bipolar. *udemy* https://www.udemy.com/course/spiritual-issues-psychosis-and-bipolar/?referralCode=FBE34891718728862D17 (2020).

36.   Withers, A. J. Disability, Divisions, Definitions, and Disablism: When Resisting Psychiatry Is Oppressive. in *Psychiatry Disrupted: Theorizing Resistance and Crafting the (R)evolution* (eds. Burstow, B., LeFrançois, B. A. & Diamond, S.) (McGill-Queen's University Press, 2014).

37.   Krishnamurti, J. When you change radically it affects all mankind. https://jkrishnamurti.org/content/when-you-change-radically-it-affects-all-mankind (1978).

38.   von Peter, S. *et al.* Open Dialogue as a Human Rights-Aligned Approach. *Front. Psychiatry* **10**, (2019).

39.   Siegel, D. J. Integration: A Central Process in the Journey to Thriving. *Garrison Institute* https://www.garrisoninstitute.org/blog/integration-a-central-process-in-the-journey-to-thriving/ (2018).

40.   Siegel, D. J. Dr. Dan Siegel on Neuroplasticity: An Excerpt from Mind. *PsychAlive* https://www.psychalive.org/dr-daniel-siegel-neuroplasticity/ (2017).

41.   Katz, D. A., Sprang, G. & Cooke, C. The cost of chronic stress in childhood: Understanding and applying the concept of allostatic load. *Psychodyn. Psychiatry* **40**, 469–480 (2012).

42.   Schioldann, J. A. What is pathography? *Med. J. Aust.* **178**, 303 (2003).

43.   Merriam-Webster. Pathography. https://www.merriam-webster.com/dictionary/pathography.

44.   Wikipedia. Post-traumatic growth. https://en.wikipedia.org/wiki/Post-traumatic_growth.

45.   Levine, P. A. & Frederick, A. *Waking the Tiger: Healing Trauma.* (North Atlantic Books, 1997).

46.   Davidson, L. The Recovery Movement: Implications for Mental Health Care and Enabling People To Participate Fully In Life. *Health Aff.* **35**, 1091–1097 (2017).

47.   Parks, J., Svendsen, D., Singer, P. & Foti, M. E. Morbidity and Mortality in

People with Serious Mental Illness N. *Natl. Assoc. State Ment. Heal. Progr. Dir.* (2006).

48. Vonnegut, M. The Eden Express: A Memoir of Insanity. (Bantam, 1975).

49. Mindell, A. City Shadows: Psychological Interventions in Psychiatry. (A. Mindell 2008)

50. Recovery in the Bin. RITB – Key Principles. https://recoveryinthebin.org/ritbkeyprinciples/ (2017).

51. Moncrieff, J. Antipsychotic Maintenance Treatment: Time to Rethink? *PLoS Med.* **12**, (2015).

52. Hengeveld, M. Job Hunting with Schizophrenia. *The Atlantic* https://www.theatlantic.com/business/archive/2015/07/job-hunting-with-schizophrenia/395936/ (2015).

53. Schwartz, M. The Possibility Principle: How Quantum Physics Can Improve the Way You Think, Live, and Love. (Sounds True, 2017).

54. Hearing Voices Network. HVN Groups Charter. https://www.hearing-voices.org/hearing-voices-groups/charter/.

55. Treatment Advocacy Center. Anosognosia. https://www.treatmentadvocacycenter.org/key-issues/anosognosia.

56. Recap Radio. A True Madness schizophrenia Documentary Real Patients. *YouTube* https://www.youtube.com/watch?v=s0NdkYs-5AU&t=2074s (2019).

57. Transdisciplinarity: Theory and Practice. (Hampton Press, 2008).

58. Cirino, E. What Are the Benefits of Hugging? *Healthline* https://www.healthline.com/health/hugging-benefits (2018).

59. Ferreira, P. R. R. The Danger of 'Normosis.' *Medium* https://medium.com/@pauloferreira8/the-danger-of-normosis-512e58383744 (2015).

60. Mcdougall, J. *Plea for A Measure of Abnormality.* (Routledge, 1993).

61. Goodreads. Aldous Huxley > Quotes. https://www.goodreads.com/quotes/94257-the-real-hopeless-victims-of-mental-illness-are-to-be.

62. Creative Maladjustment Week. Creative Maladjustment Week. http://cmweek.org/.

63. Merriam-Webster. Apophenia. https://www.merriam-webster.com/dictionary/apophenia.

64. User16591. Antonym for apophenia. *Stack Exchange* https://psychology.stackexchange.com/questions/17806/antonym-for-apophenia (2017).

65. Laing, R. D. The Politics of Experience/The Bird of Paradise. (Penguin Books, 1967).

66. Huda, S. Jaspers and un-understandability of delusions. (2019).

67. Hunter, N. Rising rates of suicide, another celebrity dead: When do we acknowledge something isn't working?! *Noel Hunter* http://www.noelrhunter.com/blogs/rising_suicide_rates/ (2018).

68. Bragdon, E. How Brazilian Spiritists Have Effectively Managed Spiritual Emergency for 100+ Years. *Spiritual Awakenings International* https://spiritualawakeningsinternational.org/event/dr-emma-bragdon-how-brazilian-spiritists-have-effectively-managed-spiritual-emergence-for-100-years/ (2021).

69. MAPS. PRESS RELEASE: Psychedelic Research Fundraising Campaign Attracts $30 Million in Donations in 6 Months, Prepares MDMA-Assisted Psychotherapy for FDA Approval. *2020* https://maps.org/news/media/8276-press-release-psychedelic-research-fundraising-campaign-attracts-$30-million-in-donations-in-6-months,-prepares-mdma-assisted-psychotherapy-for-fda-approval.

70. Wikipedia. Endocannabinoid system. https://en.wikipedia.org/wiki/Endocannabinoid_system.

71. We Plants Are Happy Plants. Terence McKenna - Consciousness Wars. *YouTube* https://www.youtube.com/watch?v=0CorHrZHHHU&t=253s (2020).

72. Berman, A. E. Are We About to Unlock the Secrets to Peak Performance? *SingularityHub* https://singularityhub.com/2017/05/14/are-we-about-to-unlock-the-secrets-to-peak-performance/ (2017).

73. The Miracle Zone. 80 % of Thoughts Are Negative…95 % are repetitive. https://faithhopeandpsychology.wordpress.com/2012/03/02/80-of-thoughts-are-negative-95-are-repetitive/ (2012).

74. Chew, S. L. Myth: We Only Use 10% of Our Brains. *Association For Psychological Science* https://www.psychologicalscience.org/teaching/myth-we-only-use-10-of-our-brains.html (2018).

75. Merriam-Webster. Meaning. https://www.merriam-webster.com/dictionary/meaning.

76. Goldhill, O. Neuroscientists can read brain activity to predict decisions 11 seconds before people act. *Quartz* https://qz.com/1569158/neuroscientists-read-unconscious-brain-activity-to-predict-decisions/ (2019).

77. Conlan, C. 5 High-Paying Jobs That Didn't Exist 10 Years Ago. *Monster* https://www.monster.com/career-advice/article/jobs-that-did-not-exist.

78. Stillpoint. Is Psychosis Meaningful? Trauma, Dissociation and

schizophrenia - Part II. *YouTube* https://www.youtube.com/watch?v=blbmeaDy21Y (2019).

79. Silberman, S. NeuroTribes: The Legacy of Autism and the Future of Neurodiversity. (Penguin Random House, 2015).

80. Bohm, D. *On Dialogue*. (Routledge, 1996).

81. Ontoscopy. Bohm: A Change of Meaning is a Change of Being. https://ontoscopy.net/extras/bohm-a-change-of-meaning-is-a-change-of-being.

82. Belair, M. 188 | Don Estes: The Science of Vibrational Sound and Light Technologies | Top Video Podcasts. *YouTube* (2018).

83. A, D. Functional neuroanatomy of altered states of consciousness: the transient hypofrontality hypothesis. *Conscious. Cogn.* **12**, 231–256 (2003).

84. Korkmaz, B. Theory of Mind and Neurodevelopmental Disorders of Childhood. *Pediatr. Res.* **69**, 101–108 (2011).

85. Brainy Quote. David Bohm Quotes. https://www.brainyquote.com/quotes/david_bohm_130977.

86. Tseng, J. & Poppenk, J. Brain meta-state transitions demarcate thoughts across task contexts exposing the mental noise of trait neuroticism. *Nat. Commun.* **11**, 1–12 (2020).

87. Neuroskeptic. The 70,000 Thoughts Per Day Myth? *Discover* https://www.discovermagazine.com/mind/the-70-000-thoughts-per-day-myth (2012).

88. Verma, P. Destroy Negativity From Your Mind With This Simple Exercise. *Medium* https://medium.com/the-mission/a-practical-hack-to-combat-negative-thoughts-in-2-minutes-or-less-cc3d1bddb3af (2017).

89. Success Chasers. 'WE ARE PROGRAMMED AT BIRTH!' - Dr. Bruce Lipton | An Eye Opening Video. *YouTube* https://www.youtube.com/watch?v=ilrj0062_zA (2019).

90. Wikipedia. Default mode network. https://en.wikipedia.org/wiki/Default_mode_network.

91. Krishnamurti, J. The Only Revolution. http://jiddu-krishnamurti.net/en/the-only-revolution/1969-00-00-jiddu-krishnamurti-the-only-revolution-india-part-1 (1969).

92. Wikipedia. Cognitive behavioral therapy. https://en.wikipedia.org/wiki/Cognitive_behavioral_therapy.

93. Tolle, E. The Power of Now: A Guide to Spiritual Enlightenment. (New World Library, 1997).

94. Humphreys, K. Tony Robbins | How To Breakthrough and Rewire Your Mind for Success with Kelsey Humphreys. *YouTube* https://www.youtube.com/watch?v=qzqAvYfYqZU&t=3019s (2016).

95. NASA. Dark Energy, Dark Matter. https://science.nasa.gov/astrophysics/focus-areas/what-is-dark-energy.

96. Mukhopadhyay, A. K. The Dynamic Web of Supracortical Consciousness. (1987).

97. vekmehel ofkirr. Bruce Lipton The Biology of Belief Full Lecture. *YouTube* https://www.youtube.com/watch?v=82ShSNuru6c&t=7723s (2014).

98. Krishnamurti, J. Follow the World Within: You Are The Story Of Humanity. (K Publications, 2015).

98b. Krishnamurti, J. The Awakening of Intelligence. (HarperSanFrancisco, 2007).

99. Wheal, J. Email from Jamie Wheal on June 24, 2021. (2021).

100. Kuil, R. Rupert Spira: Why are you so afraid of the fear? *YouTube* https://www.youtube.com/watch?v=rTe2Jb8xuJk (2015).

101. Bcassano. Seeking Awe within a Galactic Supercluster. *Medium* 2015 https://medium.com/inspire-the-world/seeking-awe-732accb44d55.

102. Akridge, J. Dolores Cannon We Are All Living Parallel Lives [FULL VIDEO]. *YouTube* https://www.youtube.com/watch?v=0re-QiF8vaU (2017).

103. Clains. On The Adjacent Possible. *Steemit* https://steemit.com/futurism/@clains/jason-silva-on-the-adjacent-possible (2016).

104. Quotefancy. Development never truly ends... https://quotefancy.com/quote/1957470/Beau-Lotto-Development-never-truly-ends-as-our-brains-evolved-to-evolve-we-are-adapted-to.

105. Redfield, J. The Celestine Vision: Living the New Spiritual Awareness. (Grand Central Publishing, 1999).

106. Doroshow, D. B. Performing a cure for schizophrenia: insulin coma therapy on the wards. *J. Hist. Med. Allied Sci.* **62**, 213–243 (2007).

107. Darchy, B., Mière, E. Le, Figuérédo, B., Bavoux, E. & Domart, Y. Iatrogenic Diseases as a Reason for Admission to the Intensive Care Unit: Incidence, Causes, and Consequences. *Arch. Intern. Med.* **159**, 71–78 (1999).

108. Cohen, D. & De Hert, M. Endogenic and iatrogenic diabetes mellitus in drug-nave schizophrenia: The role of olanzapine and its place in the psychopharmacological treatment algorithm. *Neuropsychopharmacology* **36**, 2368–2369 (2011).

109. Cuddy, A. Your body language may shape who you are. *TED* https://

www.ted.com/talks/amy_cuddy_your_body_language_may_shape_who_you_are/transcript?language=en (2012).

110. Cornwall, M. Responding to Madness with Loving Receptivity: a Practical Guide. *Mad in America* https://www.madinamerica.com/2012/02/responding-to-madness-with-loving-receptivity-a-practical-guide/ (2012).

111. Batmanghelidj, F. Your Body's Many Cries for Water: You're Not Sick; You're Thirsty: Don't Treat Thirst with Medications. (Global Health Solutions, 2008).

112. Nauert, R. Dehydration Influences Mood, Cognition. *PsychCentral* https://psychcentral.com/news/2012/02/20/dehydration-influences-mood-cognition#1 (2012).

113. Cherney, K. Effects of Bipolar Disorder on the Body. *Healthline* https://www.healthline.com/health/bipolar-disorder/effects-on-the-body (2018).

114. Ramaji & Devi, A. 1000: The Levels of Consciousness and a Map of the Stages of Awakening for Spiritual Seekers and Teachers. (Independently Published, 2019).

115. Jamison. K.R. *Touched with fire: Manic-depressive illness and the artistic temperament.* (New York: Simon & Schuster; 1996).

Made in the USA
Monee, IL
23 November 2022

18402131R00190